THE COMPLETE

WEIGHT WATCHERS COOKBOOK 2024

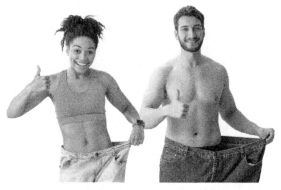

The Essential guide to healthy eating with delicious Weight Loss recipes

MARJORIE BLACK

COPYRIGHT

Disclaimer

The recipes provided in this cookbook are intended for personal use and enjoyment. While every effort has been made to ensure the accuracy of the information, the author and publisher cannot be held responsible for any errors or omissions. Cooking involves inherent risks, and readers should exercise caution and discretion when handling ingredients, appliances, and following cooking instructions.

The author and publisher disclaim any liability or responsibility for any adverse effects or consequences resulting directly or indirectly from the use of the recipes, cooking methods, or nutritional information presented in this cookbook. Individual dietary needs and health conditions vary, and readers are advised to consult with a qualified healthcare professional or nutritionist for personalized advice.

Allergen Warning: Some recipes may contain common allergens. Readers with known food allergies or sensitivities are urged to review the ingredient lists carefully and make substitutions as needed.

The nutritional information provided is an estimate and should be considered as a general guideline. Actual nutritional content may vary based on specific ingredients used and portion sizes.

By using this cookbook, readers acknowledge and agree to the terms of this disclaimer. Cooking is a creative and enjoyable activity, and individuals are encouraged to experiment and adapt recipes to suit their preferences and dietary requirements.

About the Book

"The complete Weight Watchers Cookbook," is a culinary journey through an array of delectable recipes that span various courses and culinary themes. From breakfast delights to savory dinners, each section is carefully curated to offer a diverse selection of flavors and culinary experiences.

With each recipe, I've considered not just the flavors but also the nutritional aspects, ensuring that every meal is a symphony of taste and well-being. The nutrition facts provided empower you to make informed choices while savoring the culinary delights.

"The complete Weight Watchers Cookbook" is not merely a cookbook; it is a culinary odyssey, inviting you to explore, create, and indulge in the art of cooking. May each recipe awaken your inner chef, turning every meal into a harmonious celebration of flavors. Happy cooking!

TABLE OF CONTENTS

THE COMPLETE WEIGHT WATCHERS COOKBOOK 2024

Vegan Pulled BBQ Jackfruit

INTRODUCTION

About Weight Watchers

Weight Watchers, now known as WW, is a popular and well-established weight loss and wellness program. It was founded in the 1960s by Jean Nidetch and has evolved over the years. The program focuses on a holistic approach to weight loss and overall well-being, emphasizing not just the number on the scale but also lifestyle and behavior changes.

In recent years, Weight Watchers has rebranded as WW to reflect a broader focus on overall wellness rather than just weight loss. The program continues to evolve to meet the changing needs and preferences of its members.

Key features of the Weight Watchers program include:

1. **SmartPoints System**: Foods are assigned a point value based on their nutritional content, including calories, saturated fat, sugar, and protein. Members are allocated a certain number of daily SmartPoints, and they can choose their own foods as long as they stay within their point limit.

2. **ZeroPoint Foods**: Certain healthy foods (such as fruits, vegetables, and lean proteins) have a zero SmartPoints value. This encourages members to make nutritious food choices without counting points for these items.

3. **Flexibility**: Weight Watchers promotes flexibility by allowing members to rollover unused daily SmartPoints into their weekly allowance. This flexibility accommodates social events or special occasions.

4. **Support and Community**: WW places a strong emphasis on support and community. Members can attend in-person or virtual

meetings, connect with others through the online community, and access a variety of resources, including recipes, meal plans, and fitness guidance.

5. **Wellness Focus**: Beyond weight loss, WW emphasizes overall wellness. The program encourages members to adopt healthier habits, such as regular physical activity, mindfulness, and self-care.

6. **Personalization**: WW recognizes that everyone's weight loss journey is unique. The program offers personalized plans based on individual goals, preferences, and lifestyle.

7. **Coaching and Guidance**: WW provides access to coaches who can offer personalized guidance and support to help members achieve their health and weight loss goals.

How to Use This Cookbook

Welcome to your culinary companion on the path to wellness! This section will guide you on how to make the most of the Weight Watchers New Complete Cookbook, ensuring a seamless and enjoyable cooking experience. Follow these steps to embark on a journey of delicious, health-conscious meals:

- Navigating the Recipe Pages: Each recipe is thoughtfully presented on a dedicated page, featuring a list of ingredients, clear step-by-step instructions, and the corresponding SmartPoints value. Take a moment to review the entire recipe before you begin.

- Ingredient Substitutions and Modifications: Don't hesitate to tailor recipes to suit your preferences or dietary needs. We've included tips for potential ingredient substitutions and modifications to ensure flexibility without compromising flavor or nutritional balance.

- Meal Planning and Prep Tips: Plan your meals by utilizing the meal-planning tips provided throughout the cookbook. Efficient preparation and thoughtful planning can simplify your cooking routine and contribute to a more enjoyable experience.

- Serving Suggestions and Pairings: Enhance your dining experience by exploring suggested serving sizes and complementary dishes. Discover pairing recommendations that elevate flavors and contribute to a well-rounded, satisfying meal.

- Cooking Techniques and Kitchen Essentials: Brush up on fundamental cooking techniques and essential kitchen tools mentioned in the introduction. Mastering these skills will not only make your cooking process smoother but also boost your confidence in the kitchen..

- Share and Celebrate: Connect with others on a similar wellness journey. Share your culinary creations, tips, and experiences with the Weight Watchers community. Cooking is not only about nourishing your body but also about building a supportive, inspiring network.

Tips for Successful Weight Watchers Cooking

Going on a journey toward healthier eating with Weight Watchers is not just about following recipes; it's about cultivating a mindful and sustainable approach to food. Here are some tips to enhance your success in the kitchen and make your Weight Watchers cooking experience enjoyable:

- Understand SmartPoints: Get familiar with the SmartPoints system to make informed choices. Recognize that it's not just about the number of points but the nutritional value of each ingredient.
- Meal Planning is Key: Plan your meals to avoid last-minute decisions. This helps you stay within your SmartPoints budget and ensures a well-balanced and satisfying week of eating.
- Explore Flavorful Herbs and Spices: Experiment with herbs and spices to enhance the taste of your dishes without adding extra points. Fresh herbs, garlic, ginger, and a variety of spices can transform your meals.
- Optimize Portion Control: Pay attention to portion sizes. Using smaller plates, bowls, and utensils can create the illusion of a fuller plate, helping you enjoy your meal without overeating.

- Stock a Smart Kitchen: Keep your kitchen well-stocked with nutritious staples such as whole grains, lean proteins, fresh fruits, and vegetables. Having these ingredients readily available makes it easier to create wholesome meals.

- Master Cooking Techniques: Enhance your cooking skills to make preparing meals more enjoyable. Learn techniques like roasting, grilling, and steaming to bring out natural flavors without unnecessary added fats.

- Hydration Matters: Stay hydrated! Sometimes, your body can confuse thirst for hunger. Drinking water throughout the day can help you make more mindful food choices.

- Embrace Flexibility: Be open to modifying recipes based on your preferences or dietary needs. Substitute ingredients, adjust serving sizes, and make it your own while staying mindful of SmartPoints.

- Mindful Eating Practices: Practice mindful eating by savoring each bite. Eating slowly and savoring the flavors can lead to a greater sense of satisfaction and awareness of hunger cues.

CHAPTER 1: MORNING INDULGENCE

Savory Breakfast Bowl

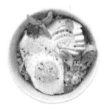 Indulge in the goodness of this versatile and easy-to-make savory breakfast bowl recipe. Feel free to customize with your favorite ingredients or make substitutions to suit your taste preferences.

Prep Time: 5 minutes

Total Time: 5 minutes

Ingredients:

- 1.5 tablespoons of high-quality extra virgin olive oil
- 6 Cherry Tomatoes (halve if large)
- A handful of Fresh Baby Spinach Leaves
- Salt, to taste
- Black pepper, to taste
- 1 cup Cooked Quinoa (prepared with salt)
- 1 Hard Boiled Egg
- 1 Small Ripe Avocado, thinly sliced
- ¼ cup Cottage Cheese
- Optional: Black Sesame Seeds

Instructions:

1. Heat olive oil in a skillet; add cherry tomatoes and spinach. Season with salt and black pepper. Sauté until spinach is wilted and cherry tomatoes are slightly cooked, approximately 2 minutes.
2. In a breakfast bowl, combine cooked quinoa (seasoned with salt), hard-boiled egg, sliced avocado, and cottage cheese.

3. Add sautéed spinach and cherry tomatoes to the bowl. Drizzle everything with olive oil and sprinkle with optional sesame seeds.
4. Enjoy this nutritious and delicious breakfast!

Notes:

- Opt for high-quality extra virgin olive oil for enhanced flavor.
- Adjust cherry tomato size as needed; halve them if they are large.
- Choose any type of quinoa available in your local store; follow package instructions for cooking time.
- Preparing ingredients the night before can save time; store eggs and quinoa in sealed containers.
- Feel free to skip sautéing cherry tomatoes and spinach; ensure proper seasoning with salt, pepper, and olive oil.

Nutrition Facts (Per Serving):

- Calories: 654kcal
- Fat: 40g
- Saturated Fat: 7g
- Cholesterol: 195mg
- Sodium: 285mg
- Potassium: 1146mg
- Carbohydrates: 54g
- Fiber: 13g
- Sugar: 7g
- Protein: 23g
- Vitamin A: 979IU
- Vitamin C: 33mg
- Calcium: 123mg
- Iron: 5mg

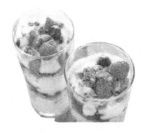

Fresh Fruit Parfaits

- Prep: 10 Minutes
- Total: 10 Minutes

Ingredients:

- ½ cup chopped cantaloupe
- ½ cup sliced strawberries
- ½ cup sliced kiwifruit or honeydew melon
- ½ banana, sliced
- 1 cup vanilla artificially sweetened low-fat yogurt
- 2 tablespoons sliced almonds, toasted

Instructions:

- Alternate layers of fruit and yogurt in 2 goblets or parfait glasses, beginning and ending with fruit.
- Top with toasted almonds.

Nutrition Facts (Per Serving):

- Calories: 160
- Total Fat: 5g
- Cholesterol: 0mg
- Sodium: 60mg
- Total Carbohydrate: 26g
- Dietary Fiber: 5g
- Protein: 8g

Nutty Banana Pancake

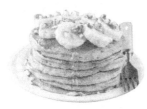

- Prep Time: 15 Minutes
- Cook Time: None (Preparation on Skillet)
- Total Time: 15 Minutes

Ingredients:

- 1 cup original pancake and baking mix
- 1/3 cup Creamy Peanut Butter
- 1 cup milk
- 1/2 large banana, chopped
- 1/2 cup pecan pieces
- 1 1/2 teaspoons ground cinnamon
- 1 large egg
- Sliced banana (for topping)
- Maple syrup (for topping)

Instructions:

- In a medium bowl, thoroughly combine pancake mix, Creamy Peanut Butter, milk, chopped banana, pecans, ground cinnamon, and egg. Ensure a well-mixed batter.
- Coat a 12-inch nonstick skillet with cooking spray and heat over medium heat.

- Scoop about 1/3 cup of batter into the skillet, spreading it evenly. Cook the pancakes, turning once, until they achieve a golden brown perfection.
- Repeat the process with the remaining batter, ensuring each pancake is cooked to golden perfection.
- Serve the pancakes topped with sliced banana and a generous drizzle of maple syrup.

Nutrition Facts (Per Serving):

- Calories per Serving: 588

CHAPTER 2: BEVERAGES And BITES

Citrus Slush Mocktail

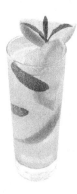

Ingredients:

- **1 ounce** lemon juice
- 1/2 ounce lime juice
- 1 1/2 ounces orange juice
- 2 ounces simple syrup
- 1 ounce water
- Fresh lime, lemon, and orange slices for garnish (optional)

Instructions:

- In a blender, combine lemon, lime, and orange juices with simple syrup and water.
- Fill the blender with ice and blend until smooth.
- Pour or spoon the slush into serving glasses.
- Garnish with twisted slices of fresh lime, lemon, and orange if desired.
- Serve and enjoy!

Mediterranean Tapenade

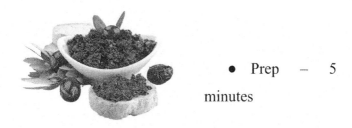

- Prep – 5 minutes

Ingredients:

- 1 cup pitted Kalamata olives
- 1 cup pitted Castelvetrano olives

- 3 oil-packed anchovy filets (optional)
- 1 large garlic clove
- 1 tablespoon water-packed capers, drained and rinsed
- 1 teaspoon chopped thyme leaves
- Black pepper
- 1 teaspoon lemon juice
- 1/4 cup extra virgin olive oil
- Zest of 1 lemon
- French baguette, cut into slices and lightly toasted (or sliced veggies)

Instructions:

- In a small food processor, combine olives, anchovy, garlic, capers, thyme, black pepper, and lemon juice. Pulse until finely chopped.
- Slowly drizzle in olive oil, pulsing until the mixture forms a runny sauce.

- Transfer olive mixture to a serving bowl, sprinkle lemon zest on top, and serve with toasted bread or veggies.

Nutrition Facts (Per Serving):

- Calories: 112.9kcal
- Carbohydrates: 1.6g
- Protein: 0.8g
- Fat: 12.1gSaturated Fat:
- Cholesterol: 1.3mg
- Sugar: 0.2g

Spinach Artichoke Dip

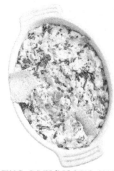

Ingredients:

- 8 ounces cream cheese, softened
- 2/3 cup sour cream
- 1/3 cup mayonnaise
- 2 cloves garlic, minced
- 1 1/2 cups shredded mozzarella cheese
- 1/2 cup shredded parmesan cheese
- 1/2 cup shredded Gruyere cheese
- 10 ounces frozen chopped spinach, thawed and squeezed dry
- 14 ounces marinated artichoke hearts, drained and chopped

Instructions:

- Preheat the oven to 375°F.
- In a bowl, beat cream cheese, sour cream, mayonnaise, and garlic until fluffy.
- Gently fold in mozzarella, parmesan, Gruyere, spinach, and artichokes.

- Spread the mixture in a 9x9 casserole dish, top with mozzarella cheese, and bake until bubbly and browned.
- Let it rest for 10 minutes before serving. Enjoy with tortilla chips, baguette slices, crackers, or veggies.

Tips:

- Utilize a hand mixer for a dip with a softer, smoother texture.
- Rapidly thaw spinach by placing it in a fine mesh strainer and rinsing it under hot water.
- Employ your hands or a spoon to gently squeeze or press the spinach, extracting any excess moisture.
- If you prefer fresh spinach over frozen, cook 1lb of spinach, cool, squeeze dry, chop, and use as directed.

- Plan by preparing this dip up to 48 hours before serving and bake it just before presenting. If refrigerated, it might need an additional 5 minutes to cook thoroughly.

Nutrition Facts (Per Serving):

- Calories: 292
- Carbohydrates: 15g
- Protein: 12g
- Fat: 20g
- Cholesterol: 42mg
- Sugar: 2g

CHAPTER 3: SALAD: SIDES AND MAIN DISHES

Grilled Caesar Salad

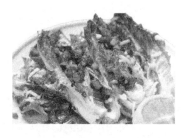

Ingredients:

- 1 large egg yolk (see Tip)
- 2 anchovy fillets, finely chopped to a paste (about 1 1/2 teaspoons)
- ½ teaspoon Dijon mustard
- ½ teaspoon grated garlic
- ½ teaspoon Worcestershire sauce
- ¼ teaspoon salt
- 2 ounces Parmesan cheese, grated with a microplane (about 1 1/4 cups), divided

- ⅓ cup mild olive oil plus 2 tablespoons, divided
- 2 heads romaine lettuce, outer leaves removed, halved lengthwise through root
- 1 medium lemon, halved crosswise
- 4 (1-inch-thick) slices whole-grain bread

Instructions:

- Whisk egg yolk, anchovy, mustard, garlic, Worcestershire, salt, and 1/4 cup Parmesan together in a medium bowl until well combined. Whisking constantly, gradually add 1/3 cup oil. Cover and refrigerate until ready to use.
- Preheat a gas grill to high (about 450°F to 500°F). Arrange romaine halves and lemon halves, cut sides up, on a large baking sheet. Drizzle with the remaining 2 tablespoons of oil and set aside.

- Place bread on unoiled grates; grill, uncovered, until charred and crispy, 1 to 2 minutes per side. Transfer to a cutting board and set aside.
- Place romaine halves and lemons, cut-sides down, on unoiled grates; grill, uncovered, turning lettuce once halfway, until the lettuce is lightly charred on both sides and the cut sides of the lemons are charred 2 to 4 minutes. Remove from the grill; place romaine on a cutting board and slice in half lengthwise (making 8 wedges total).
- Cut the charred bread into bite-size pieces. Juice 1 lemon half into the dressing mixture and whisk to combine.
- Arrange the romaine wedges on a platter; drizzle with half the dressing mixture (about 1/4 cup) and top with the croutons. Juice the remaining lemon half over the salad. Sprinkle with the remaining 1 cup

Parmesan. Serve immediately, with the remaining dressing.

Tips:

When a recipe calls for raw eggs, you can minimize the risk of foodborne illness by using pasteurized-in-the-shell eggs. Look for them in the refrigerator case near other whole eggs.

Mango Avocado Tango

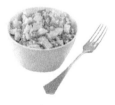

This creation was born during an unexpected blackout at a blogger conference, where chefs from the California Avocado Commission challenged participants to craft inventive guacamoles by candlelight.

Ingredients:

- 4 Hass avocados
- 1/2 cup diced mango
- 1/2 cup diced pineapple
- 1/2 cup minced red onion
- 1/2 cup finely chopped cilantro
- 1/2 cup diced tomatoes
- 1/3 cup diced cucumber
- 1 teaspoon red pepper flakes
- 1/3 cup dried cherries
- Juice of 1 lemon
- 2 tablespoons rice vinegar
- Salt to taste

Instructions:

- In a medium bowl, mash the avocados.
- Add mango, pineapple, red onion, cilantro, tomatoes, cucumber, red pepper flakes, dried cherries, lemon juice, rice vinegar, and salt. Mix well.
- Taste for seasoning and adjust as needed.
- Serve and enjoy the tropical burst of flavors in every bite!

CHAPTER 4: MAIN DISHES

A. Starters

i. Caprese Bruschetta

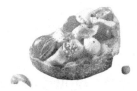

Ingredients:

- Ripe tomatoes (hot house, tomatoes on the vine, heirloom, etc.)
- Kosher salt
- High-quality extra-virgin olive oil
- Garlic cloves, minced
- Red pepper flakes
- Mozzarella pearls
- Fresh basil leaves
- Freshly ground black pepper

- Balsamic glaze
- Crusty bread (ciabatta or French baguette)

Instructions:

- Preheat the oven to 350°F and line a baking sheet.
- Chop tomatoes and let them drain in a colander with salt for 20 minutes.
- In a skillet, heat olive oil with garlic and red pepper flakes until fragrant; let it cool.
- Brush both sides of bread slices with garlic oil and bake until golden.
- Combine drained tomatoes with mozzarella, garlic oil, basil, salt, and pepper.
- Top toasted bread slices with the bruschetta mixture, drizzle with balsamic glaze and serve.

Make-Ahead:

- Prepare elements up to a day ahead, store ingredients separately, toast the bread before serving, and assemble just before serving.

Serving Suggestions:

- Pair with marinated olives, prosciutto-wrapped melon, or an antipasto platter for a complete Italian-themed experience.

Storage:

- Best enjoyed the day of making; however, store the tomato-cheese mixture separately from the bread for up to 2 days

Tips:

- Ensure tomatoes drain to prevent bread sogginess.
- Opt for balsamic glaze for a thicker and sweeter alternative to vinegar.
- For a dairy-free version, omit the cheese or substitute with avocado a creamy element
- Utilize a hand mixer for a dip with a softer, smoother texture.
- Rapidly thaw spinach by placing it in a fine mesh strainer and rinsing it under hot water.
- Employ your hands or a spoon to gently squeeze or press the spinach, extracting any excess moisture.
- If you prefer fresh spinach over frozen, cook 1lb of spinach, cool, squeeze dry, chop, and use as directed.
- Plan by preparing this dip up to 48 hours before serving and bake it just before presenting. If refrigerated, it might need an additional 5 minutes to cook thoroughly.

Nutrition Facts (Per Serving):

- Calories: 292
- Carbohydrates: 15g
- Protein: 12g
- Fat: 20g
- Cholesterol: 42mg
- Sugar: 2g

ii. Lemon Garlic Shrimp Skewers

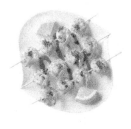

For a healthy protein option, consider our Lemon Garlic Shrimp Skewers. Marinated in fresh garlic, lemon, and white wine, these skewers make a perfect addition to any meal. Low in fat and bursting with flavor, these shrimp skewers are versatile, and suitable for salads, wraps, or pairing with roasted potatoes and grilled veggies.

Shrimp Skewer:

- Skewers (metal or bamboo)
- Low baking dish
- Whisk
- Mixing bowl
- Grill (indoor or outdoor)

Ingredients:

- Shrimp
- Lemon
- Olive oil
- Garlic cloves
- White wine
- Dried parsley

- Salt
- Pepper
- Parsley (for garnish)

Instructions:

- Soak skewers in water.
- Whisk together lemon zest, lemon juice, olive oil, garlic, white wine, parsley, salt, and pepper.
- Rinse and prepare shrimp, skewering them.
- Marinate shrimp in the prepared mixture for 20-30 minutes.
- Grill skewers on low heat until shrimp turns pink and opaque.

Nutrition Facts (Per Serving):

- Calories: 54kcal

- Fat: 5g
- Sodium: 3mg
- Carbohydrates: 1g
- Fiber: 1g
- Sugar: 1g
- Protein: 1g
- Vitamin C: 1mg
- Calcium: 5mg
- Iron: 1mg

B. Beef & Lamb

i. Rosemary Garlic Beef Tenderloin

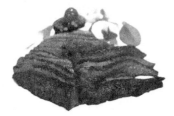

- Prep Time: 10 minutes
- Cook Time: 45 minutes
- Resting Time: 10 minutes

- Total Time: 1 hour 5 minutes

Ingredients:

- 1/2 tablespoon extra virgin olive oil
- 4 cloves garlic, minced
- 1 tablespoon fresh rosemary, chopped
- 1 tablespoon Kosher salt, and freshly ground black pepper, to taste
- 1 4-pound beef tenderloin, trimmed and tied into 2-inch sections

Instructions:

- Preheat oven to 375 degrees F. Line a baking sheet with foil and coat with oil spray.
- In a small bowl, combine olive oil, garlic, rosemary, salt, and black pepper.

- Pat tenderloin dry with paper towels. Season all over with garlic mixture, gently pressing to adhere.
- Place tenderloin onto the prepared baking sheet. Bake until it reaches an internal temperature of 125 to 130 degrees F for medium-rare, about 45 minutes to 1 hour, or until desired doneness.
- Let the beef rest for 10 minutes before slicing.
- Serve immediately.

Nutrition Facts (Per Serving):

- Calories: 211 kcal
- Carbohydrates: 0.5 g
- Protein: 33.5 g
- Fat: 8.5 g
- Saturated Fat: 2.5 g
- Cholesterol: 93.5 mg

- Sodium: 343.5 mg

Serving Suggestions:

- Vegetables: Parmesan Brussels Sprouts, Grilled Asparagus, Roasted Mushrooms
- Starches: Baked Potatoes, Garlic Mashed Potatoes, Rice Pilaf
- Holiday Side Dishes: Cornbread Stuffing, Green Bean Casserole, Spinach Gratin
- Sandwiches: Roast Beef Sandwich with Swiss and Onions, Roast Beef, Arugula, and Parmesan on Baguette

Storage:

- Store leftover beef in the refrigerator for up to four days and reheat it in the microwave until warm.

ii. Minted Lamb Chops

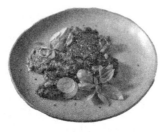

- Prep Time: 10 minutes
- Cook Time: 8 minutes

Ingredients:

- 4 pieces of Lamb Chops
- 6-8 pieces of Mint Leaves
- 2 tbsp Olive Oil
- 1 clove Garlic, chopped
- 1 piece Shallot, chopped

Instructions:

- Add the shallot, mint, olive oil, and garlic to a food processor. Mix until ingredients become a paste.
- Spread the mint paste over the lamb chops using a spoon.
- In a medium-heated grill pan or frying pan, add a little bit of oil. Add the lamb chops with the mint paste side down and let them cook for about 4 minutes.
- Spread the remaining paste on the other side of the meat before flipping. Cook for another 4 minutes.

How to Serve:

- Pair with roasted vegetables like potatoes, carrots, and parsnips, or a colorful salad with a light vinaigrette.

- For a heartier option, serve with mashed potatoes or roasted potatoes, steamed broccoli, or green beans.
- For a decadent dish, pair with grilled asparagus and crumbled feta cheese.

How to Know When Lamb Chops are Done:

- Use a meat thermometer for accuracy. For medium-rare, aim for an internal temperature of 145°F.

Storage:

- Cool lamb chops to room temperature before refrigerating. Wrap in aluminum foil or store in an airtight container.
- Consume within three to four days.

Nutrition Facts (Per Serving):

- Energy: 433 kcal
- Total Fat: 13.5 g
- Saturates: 4.2 g
- Carbs: 39.4 g
- Sugars: 7.2 g
- Fiber: 5.1 g
- Protein: 35.8 g
- Salt: 0.3 g

C. Seafoods Symphony

i. Salmon with Citrus Glaze

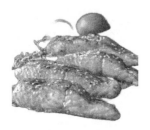

- Prep Time: 5 minutes
- Cook Time: 20 minutes
- Total Time: 25 minutes

Ingredients:

- **Citrus Sauce or Glaze**:
  - 1 orange (zest and juice)

- 1 small lime (zest and juice)
- 1/2 lemon (zest and juice)
- 3 tablespoons maple syrup or honey or brown sugar (or more to taste)
- 2 teaspoons Dijon mustard
- 1/2 teaspoon cornstarch (optional)

- **Salmon:**
  - 1 pound salmon fillets (one larger filet or 2-3 individual fillets)
  - Salt and black pepper
  - 2 green onions, chopped

- **Garnish options:**
  - Lime wedges for squeezing

Instructions:

- Preheat the oven or toaster oven to 425F/218C. Line a baking sheet with parchment paper or aluminum foil sprayed with oil.

- **Make Glaze**: In a small saucepan, combine orange-lime-lemon zest, orange juice, lemon-lime juice, maple syrup, Dijon mustard, a pinch of salt, and red pepper flakes (if using).
- Bring to a boil, then simmer for 5-7 minutes until the mixture thickens slightly. Taste and adjust as needed.
- **Prepare Salmon**: Place salmon fillets on the prepared pan, skin side down.
- Sprinkle salmon with salt and pepper.
- Brush a couple of tablespoons of glaze over the salmon.
- Sprinkle chopped green onions.
- Roast for 10-12 minutes, depending on thickness. Brush on more glaze halfway through.
- Remove the skin by sliding a spatula between the skin and the salmon meat.
- Drizzle the remaining glaze over the salmon.
- Garnish as desired with lime wedges.

- Serve hot, at room temperature, or cold.

Notes:

- For the glaze, you can use any combination of citrus fruits, add chopped cilantro, and red pepper flakes for heat, or stir in cold butter for a velvety finish.
- Salmon can be substituted with other mild fish like snapper, halibut, trout, or perch fillets.

Nutrition Facts (Per Serving):

- Protein: 47 g
- Fat: 15 g
- Calories: 459 kcal
- Cholesterol: 125 mg
- Sodium: 455 mg

- Carbohydrates: 35 g
- Sugar: 26 g
- Saturated Fat: 2 g
- Potassium: 1402 mg
- Fiber: 4 g
- Vitamin A: 395 IU
- Vitamin C: 61 mg
- Calcium: 113 mg
- Iron: 2 mg

ii. Shrimp and Scallop Scampi

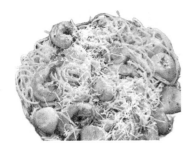

- Prep Time: 15 minutes
- Cook Time: 15 minutes
- Total Time: 30 minutes

Ingredients:

- 1/2 cup extra-virgin olive oil
- 3 large cloves garlic, minced
- 1/3 cup red onion, thinly sliced
- Salt to taste
- 1 tablespoon red pepper flakes
- 1 pound medium-sized shrimp, peeled and deveined
- 6 ounces bay scallops
- 1 cup sweet mini pepper, thinly sliced
- 1/2 cup white wine
- 2 tablespoons freshly squeezed lemon juice
- 3 tablespoons butter
- Chopped fresh parsley leaves
- Freshly ground black pepper
- Grated Parmesan cheese for serving

Instructions:

- Heat olive oil in a large skillet over medium heat. Add garlic and red onion, followed by a pinch of salt. Cook slowly until fragrant.
- Add red pepper flakes.
- Switch heat to medium-high, add shrimp, scallops, and sweet mini pepper. Cook until the seafood is almost done (about 4-5 minutes). Stir occasionally.
- Add white wine, fresh lemon juice, and butter. Cook for another minute or until the butter is melted in the sauce. Taste, and add more salt if needed.
- Serve over pasta with the scampi sauce. Top with chopped fresh parsley leaves, a grind of black pepper, and grated Parmesan cheese. Enjoy!

Nutrition Facts (Per Serving):

- Protein: 32.4g

- Total Fat: 38g
- Calories: 487
- Cholesterol: 222.8mg
- Sodium: 422.1mg
- Carbohydrates: 7.4g
- Sugar: 2.5g
- Saturated Fat: 9.6g
- Fiber: 1.4g

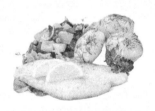

iii. Grilled Halibut with Mango Salsa

- Prep Time: 15 minutes
- Cook Time: 10 minutes
- Total Time: 25 minutes

Ingredients:

- **For the Salsa**:
    - 1 large ripe mango, diced
    - ½ small red onion, diced
    - ¼ cup fresh cilantro, chopped
    - 1 medium red bell pepper, diced
    - 2 tbsp lime juice (about 2 small limes)
    - ¼ tsp salt
- **For the Fish**:
    - 1 lb halibut filet
    - 1 tbsp olive oil
    - ½ tsp black pepper
- **To Garnish**:
    - Lime wedges for squeezing

Instructions:

- **Mango Salsa**:
    - In a medium mixing bowl, combine all salsa ingredients and mix well.

- Optional: Let it marinate for 10+ minutes for enhanced flavors.

- **Prepare and Grill Halibut**:
  - Pat the fish dry and season both sides with salt and pepper.
  - Heat a grill or pan over medium heat and add oil.
  - Cook the fish for 4-6 minutes per side until opaque throughout. The time depends on thickness (rule of thumb: 10 minutes per inch).
  - Brush with olive oil during cooking and halfway through.

- **Finish and Serve**:
  - Let the fish rest for a minute or two before garnishing with the salsa.
  - Store extra salsa in an airtight container for future use.

Notes:

- For the salsa, be sure the mango is ripe for optimal flavor.
- Additional garnish options: chopped fresh parsley, black pepper, and a squeeze of lime.
- Clean and oil the grill grates for easy cooking and prevent sticking.

Nutrition Facts (Per Serving):

- Protein: 47g
- Total Fat: 15g

- Calories: 363
- Cholesterol: 125mg
- Sodium: 455mg
- Carbohydrates: 35g
- Sugar: 26g
- Iron: 2mg
- Calcium: 113mg
- Potassium: 1402mg
- Fiber: 4g
- Vitamin A: 395IU
- Vitamin C: 61mg

D. Poultry Pleasures

i. Lemon Herb Roasted Chicken

- Prep Time: 10 mins
- Cook Time: 30 mins

- Total Time: 40 mins

Ingredients:

- 1 chicken, cut into 10 pieces
- 1/4 cup lemon juice
- 2 tbsp extra virgin olive oil
- 1 tbsp minced garlic
- 3/4 tsp salt
- 3/4 tsp black pepper
- 1 tbsp fresh rosemary, chopped
- 1 tbsp fresh oregano, chopped
- 2 lemons, cut into thin circles
- Optional: a little extra fresh herbs to add after baking

Instructions:

- Preheat the oven to 450 degrees.

- Spread the chicken on a baking sheet (use a 9 x 13 sheet or larger if needed).
- In a bowl, combine all other ingredients except the lemon slices. Stir and pour over the chicken.
- Add lemon slices on top of and/or in between the chicken pieces on the baking sheet.
- Place in the oven and bake for 30 minutes. Remove from the oven.
- Spoon some pan gravy and an extra pinch of fresh herbs onto the chicken as you plate it.

Nutrition Facts (Per Serving):

- Calories: 329 kcal
- Carbohydrates: 4 g
- Protein: 24 g
- Fat: 23 g
- Cholesterol: 95 mg

- Sodium: 380 mg
- Potassium: 300 mg
- Fiber: 1 g
- Sugar: 1 g
- Vitamin A: 180 IU
- Vitamin C: 25.5 mg
- Calcium: 26 mg
- Iron: 1.4 mg

ii. Coconut Chicken Curry

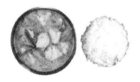

- Prep Time: 5 mins
- Cook Time: 25 mins
- Total Time: 30 mins

Ingredients:

- 2 tbsp olive oil
- 2 lbs chicken breasts, skinless and boneless, cut into bite-size pieces
- ½ tsp salt (or to taste)
- ½ tsp pepper (or to taste)
- 1 small onion, chopped
- 3 cloves garlic, minced
- 2 tbsp curry powder
- 1 cup chicken broth (low sodium)
- 14 oz coconut milk (1 can)
- 14.5 oz diced tomatoes (1 can)
- 2 tbsp tomato paste
- 2 tbsp sugar
- 2 tbsp parsley, chopped

Instructions:

- Heat olive oil in a large skillet or Dutch oven. Add chicken, season with salt and pepper, and cook until no longer pink.

- Add onion, garlic, curry powder, and stir. Cook for 2 more minutes, then add chicken broth, coconut milk, tomatoes, tomato paste, and sugar. Stir and bring to a boil. Cover with a lid, reduce heat, and simmer for 15 to 20 minutes.
- Garnish with parsley and serve over rice.

Storage:

- Leftovers can be stored in an airtight container and refrigerated for 5 days. For longer storage, freeze curry and rice separately in freezer-safe containers for up to 2 months.

Nutrition Facts (Per Serving):

- Calories: 396 kcal

- Carbohydrates: 13 g
- Protein: 35 g
- Fat: 23 g
- Saturated Fat: 14 g
- Cholesterol: 97 mg
- Sodium: 532 mg
- Potassium: 977 mg
- Fiber: 2 g
- Sugar: 7 g
- Vitamin C: 12 mg
- Calcium: 58 mg
- Iron: 4 mg

F. Vegetarian Varieties

i. Eggplant Parmesan Stacks

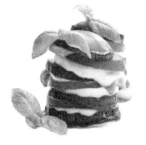

- Prep Time: 1 hour 5 minutes
- Cooking Time: 15 minutes
- Final Dish Cook: 20 minutes
- Total Time: 1 hour 40 minutes

Ingredients:

Salting the Eggplant

- 2 eggplants, sliced into ⅓" slices (approximately 8 slices per eggplant)
- 2 tsp kosher salt (1 teaspoon per sheet pan for salting the eggplant)

Breading

- ¼ cup flour
- 3 large eggs, beaten
- ½ cup grated Parmesan cheese
- ½ cup panko
- ½ cup seasoned Italian breadcrumbs
- 8 slices fresh mozzarella, cut/torn in half
- 3½ cups Italian tomato sauce (either Easy Tomato Sauce or Italian Red Sauce, or about 3 ½ cups of your favorite tomato sauce)

Ricotta Filling

- 15 oz whole milk ricotta
- 1 large egg, lightly beaten
- ½ cup grated Parmesan cheese
- 1 teaspoon lemon zest
- 1 teaspoon kosher salt

- ½ teaspoon pepper (or 2 teaspoons dried)
- 2 tablespoons fresh flat-leaf Italian parsley, chopped
- ½ cup grated mozzarella (optional)

Instructions:

Salting

- Slice the eggplants into approximately 8 slices each, ⅓" thick.
- Arrange 8 eggplant slices on a baking sheet covered with two layers of paper towels. Repeat on a second sheet.
- Sprinkle 1 teaspoon of salt in each pan and let the eggplant rest for 1 hour.
- After 1 hour, lightly rinse the eggplant and pat dry with a paper towel.

Breading

- Preheat the oven to 400°F. Grease a baking sheet with 1 tablespoon of olive oil or baking spray.
- Place flour in a shallow dish, beat eggs in a wide shallow pie plate, and combine breadcrumbs and cheese in another shallow dish.
- Dip each side of the eggplant slices in flour, then beaten eggs, and finally the breadcrumb mixture. Transfer to the prepared baking sheet.
- Bake for 15-18 minutes, flipping halfway through, until crispy. Adjust time-based on your oven.
- Allow the baked slices to cool.

Assemble

- Pour one cup of tomato sauce into a 9x13" pan.
- Layer half of the eggplant slices on the sauce.
- Top with half a piece of fresh mozzarella and a generous tablespoon of sauce. Repeat.
- Spoon another tablespoon of sauce and a large dollop of ricotta filling onto the top of each eggplant tower.
- Sprinkle-grated mozzarella or Parmesan on top if using.
- Bake in a 400°F oven for 20 minutes until the cheese is melted.

Notes:

- **Options**: Layer prosciutto between the stacks or add cooked crumbled Italian sausage and ground beef to the sauce for a meat version.

- **Make ahead**: Prep and bread the eggplant slices earlier in the day, refrigerate, and follow baking and assembly directions an hour before serving.
- The ricotta mixture can be made a couple of days in advance.
- Utilize any frozen or available sauce.
- For an air fryer (1-3 servings), follow the provided instructions after breading the eggplant.

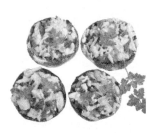

ii. Spinach And Ricotta Stuffed Portobello Mushrooms

- Prep Time: 15 minutes
- Cook Time: 25 minutes

Ingredients:

- 3 medium portobello mushrooms, stemmed and gills scraped out
- 2 cups fresh spinach
- 1/2 cup water
- 1/2 cup red bell pepper, diced small
- 1/3 cup diced onion (small dice)
- 1 cup part-skim ricotta cheese
- 1/4 cup grated Parmesan cheese
- 1 cup shredded mozzarella, divided
- 1 tsp fresh garlic, minced
- 2 slices bacon, cooked & crumbled (optional)

Instructions:

- Preheat the oven to 425°F. Cover a baking sheet with foil and lightly spray with non-cooking spray. Place mushrooms, gill side up, on the baking sheet.

- In a small skillet, add spinach with 1/2 cup water, cover, and cook on medium-high heat until spinach has wilted. Drain well and squeeze to remove any excess water. Set aside.
- Combine ricotta, Parmesan, and 3/4 cup mozzarella in a medium-sized bowl.
- Add bell pepper, onion, garlic, and spinach to the cheese mixture. Combine well.
- If using bacon, mix it in.
- Stuff mushrooms with the cheese mixture.
- Top with remaining mozzarella.
- Bake for approximately 25 minutes.

CHAPTER 5: SMALL PLATES SYMPHONY

1. Mini Veggie Pizzas

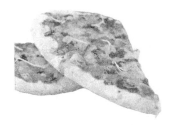

- Preparation Time: 20 minutes
- Cooking Time: 10 minutes
- Total Time: 30 minutes

Ingredients:

- 1 large zucchini, halved lengthwise
- 1 red bell pepper, halved
- 1 tablespoon olive oil
- 1 cup marinara sauce (e.g., Rao's)

- 1 package (6-count) whole wheat pita bread rounds
- 1 block (8 oz) part-skim mozzarella cheese, shredded
- ½ cup thinly sliced red onion
- ½ cup halved pitted kalamata olives
- ½ cup crumbled feta cheese
- 2 tablespoons chopped fresh basil

Instructions:

- Preheat the grill to medium-high heat.
- Toss zucchini and bell pepper with olive oil and grill, covered, for 5 minutes or until tender.
- Cut zucchini into ¼-inch slices and bell pepper into strips.
- Spread marinara sauce on pitas; top with mozzarella, onion, olives, grilled vegetables, and feta.

- Grill, covered, for 2 to 3 minutes or until cheese is melted and pitas are crisp.
- Sprinkle with chopped basil.

Nutrition Facts (Per Serving):

- Calories: 392
- Fat (g): 19
- Sat Fat (g): 7
- Protein (g): 18
- Carb (g): 39
- Fiber (g): 4
- Sodium (mg): 899

2. Stuffed Mushrooms Trio

i. Sausage-Stuffed Mushroom:

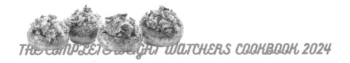

- **Ingredients**:
  - 24 crimini mushrooms (stems and gills removed)
  - 12 oz ground Italian sausage
  - 8 oz cream cheese, softened and cubed
  - 2 cups diced yellow onions
  - 5 garlic cloves, minced
  - 1 tsp red chili flakes
  - 6 oz shredded parmesan
  - Salt and Pepper (to taste)

Instructions:

- Sauté onions, garlic, and ground sausage until cooked. Add chili flakes.
- Combine sausage mixture with cream cheese and parmesan.
- Fill each mushroom with the mixture and roast for 14 minutes at 350 degrees.

ii. Feta and Spinach Stuffed Mushroom:

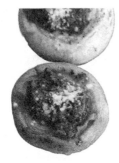

Ingredients:

- 24 crimini mushrooms (stems and gills removed)
- 8 oz chopped spinach, thawed
- 4 oz cream cheese
- 8 oz feta cheese
- ½ cup finely chopped green onions
- ½ tsp garlic salt
- ½ tsp black pepper
- 1 cup grated parmesan

Instructions:

- Combine all ingredients (except mushrooms) in a mixing bowl.
- Fill each mushroom with the spinach mixture, sprinkle parmesan on top, and roast for 14 minutes at 350 degrees.

iii. Crab Stuffed Mushrooms:

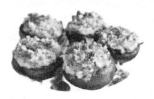

Ingredients:

- 24 crimini mushrooms (stems and gills removed)
- 8 oz cream cheese
- ¼ cup grated parmesan
- 3 tbsp sour cream
- 3 tbsp mayonnaise
- 1 tbsp Worcestershire sauce
- 1 tsp Tabasco or hot sauce
- 1 tsp Old Bay seasoning

- Zest and juice of 1 lemon
- 2 tbsp chives
- 2 tbsp chopped fresh parsley
- 8 oz jumbo crab meat

Instructions:

- Whisk together all ingredients (except crab) in a mixing bowl.
- Gently fold in crab meat and spoon the mixture into mushrooms.
- Roast for 14 minutes at 350 degrees.

3. Tomato Chutney

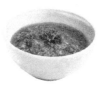

Ingredients:

- 8 tomatoes
- 2 tbsp vegetable oil
- 2 green chilies, seeds removed, finely chopped
- 1 tsp cumin
- 1 tsp mustard powder
- ½ tsp turmeric
- 1 tsp mild chili powder
- 2 garlic cloves, finely chopped or grated
- ¼ tsp salt
- ½ tsp granulated sugar
- 1 bay leaf
- Fresh cilantro, chopped

Instructions:

- Score an X on the bottom of the tomatoes and simmer in hot water for 5 minutes. Peel and chop.

- In a sauté pan, cook cumin, mustard powder, turmeric, chili powder, chilies, and garlic.
- Stir in tomatoes, salt, sugar, and bay leaf. Simmer for 10 minutes covered, then 5 more minutes uncovered.
- Serve garnished with fresh cilantro.

Nutritional Facts (Per Serving):

- Calories: 63
- Total Fat: 4g
- Cholesterol: 0mg
- Sodium: 84mg
- Carbohydrates: 7g
- Fiber: 2g
- Sugar: 4g
- Protein: 2g

CHAPTER 6 GRILL MASTER'S COLLECTION

Grilled Vegetable Platter

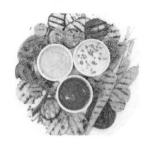

Ingredients:

- 2 zucchinis, sliced into ½-1 inch slices
- 8 ounces cremini mushrooms (skewered for grilling)
- 8–10 mini bell peppers, left whole (or 2 medium bell peppers, sliced into 4–5 flat planks)
- 8 ounces grape tomatoes, left whole (skewered for grilling)

- 4 shallots, peeled and halved lengthwise with ends intact
- ½-1 lbs asparagus spears, woody ends trimmed
- 5 tablespoons olive oil
- 2 tablespoons balsamic vinegar
- 1 teaspoon salt
- ¼ teaspoon pepper
- 1 ½ teaspoons dried Italian seasoning
- 2 cloves of garlic, peeled and minced

Chimichurri Sauce Ingredients:

- ¼ cup packed parsley leaves & tender stems, finely chopped
- 1 heaping tablespoon packed fresh oregano leaves, finely chopped
- 2 cloves garlic, peeled and minced
- 5 tablespoons extra virgin olive oil
- 1 tablespoon balsamic vinegar

- ½ teaspoon crushed red pepper flake
- ½ teaspoon each salt and ground black pepper or to taste

For Serving (optional):

- Grilled bread
- Ricotta or burrata

Instructions:

- Begin by making the chimichurri sauce. Combine all the chimichurri ingredients in a jar or container with a tight lid. Shake well, then refrigerate until ready to use.
- In a large bowl, whisk together olive oil, balsamic vinegar, salt, pepper, dried Italian seasoning, and minced garlic.

- Add the prepared vegetables to the bowl and toss them to coat thoroughly. Cover and refrigerate for at least 20 minutes to 2 hours for marination.
- Preheat your grill or grill pan to medium-high heat. Grease the grill grates.
- Skewer smaller veggies like mushrooms and grape tomatoes for easier grilling.
- Grill the vegetables over medium-high heat for 3-5 minutes per side or until browned and tender.
- Serve the grilled vegetables on a platter, drizzle generously with chimichurri sauce, and optionally pair with grilled bread and ricotta or burrata.
- Enjoy the grilled vegetables either warm or at room temperature.

Grilled Vegetable Pairing Ideas:

- Grilled potatoes
- Grilled Greek Chicken
- Pesto pasta
- Grilled steak, pork, or any protein
- Use in sandwiches, wraps, or flatbreads

Storage Tip:

- Leftover grilled vegetables can be stored in an airtight container in the fridge for 2-4 days. Enjoy them cold, at room temperature, or reheated in the microwave or on the stove.

How to Grill Vegetables for Maximum Flavor:

- **Prepare the Marinade/Dressing**:
    - Mix ingredients like olive oil, balsamic vinegar, herbs, and spices

for a flavorful marinade or dressing. Some prefer to dress veggies after grilling, while others marinate before cooking.

- Coat the veggies thoroughly in the marinade. For enhanced flavor, marinate them for a few hours or even overnight.
- Preheat your grill to medium-high heat, typically around 350-400°F.
- For smaller veggies like cherry tomatoes or mushrooms, consider skewering for easy grilling.
- Ensure well-oiled grill grates to prevent sticking and achieve those coveted grill marks.
- Grill the vegetables over medium-high heat until tender with a slight char. The cooking time varies, so keep an eye on them, turning occasionally.

- Arrange the grilled vegetables on a platter, and drizzle with additional marinade or dressing for maximum flavor.
- Grilled vegetables are versatile and perfect for topping burgers and sandwiches, or adding to salads. Enjoy them as a side dish or incorporate them into various recipes for a burst of smoky goodness.

Teriyaki Chicken Pineapple Kabobs

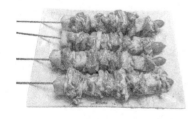

Teriyaki Sauce Marinade:

- ¼ cup low-sodium soy sauce

- 3 tablespoons brown sugar
- 1 clove garlic, minced
- 1 teaspoon fresh ginger, grated (or ¼ teaspoon ground ginger)
- Pinch of salt and black pepper
- 1 tablespoon cornstarch
- 1 tablespoon water

Kabob Ingredients:

- 2 lbs. boneless, skinless chicken breasts, cut into 1-inch cubes
- 1 lb. package of cooked turkey rope sausage, cut into 1-inch chunks
- 1 ½ cups fresh pineapple, cut into 1-inch cubes
- 1 small red bell pepper, cut into 1-inch chunks
- 1 small green bell pepper, cut into 1-inch chunks

- ½ medium red onion cut into 1-inch chunks

Instructions:

- Craft the teriyaki marinade: In a small saucepan, combine soy sauce, brown sugar, minced garlic, grated ginger, salt, and black pepper. Bring to a boil, then reduce heat, simmer for 1-2 minutes until slightly thickened, and let it cool. Reserve about 3 tablespoons for basting and dipping.
- Place chicken pieces in a ziplock bag, add the teriyaki marinade (excluding the reserved part), and toss to coat. Marinate for at least 30 minutes (2 hours for optimal flavor).
- Soak wooden skewers in water for 30 minutes to prevent burning during grilling.
- Preheat the grill.

- Assemble the kabobs by threading marinated chicken, pineapple, sausage, red and green bell peppers, and red onion onto the soaked skewers.
- Grill over medium heat for 10-12 minutes, turning occasionally, until the chicken is cooked through, sausage is warmed, and vegetables are tender.
- Brush with the reserved teriyaki sauce during the last moments of grilling or serve on the side for dipping.

Note: Experiment with different combinations of chicken and sausage or opt for veggie-only kabobs for diverse preferences.

Nutrition Facts (Per Serving):

- Calories: 372
- Total Fat: 11g

- Saturated Fat: 3g
- Trans Fat: 0g
- Unsaturated Fat: 6g
- Cholesterol: 163mg
- Sodium: 518mg
- Carbohydrates: 12g
- Fiber: 1g
- Sugar: 9g
- Protein: 54g

CHAPTER 7: GRAIN AND PASTA SIDE DISHES

Lemon-Basil Orzotto

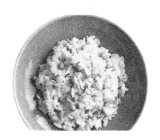

Ingredients:

- 2 tablespoons extra-virgin olive oil
- 1 cup diced onion
- 1 1/2 cups orzo or pearl barley
- 1/2 cup dry white wine
- 3 cups chicken stock or low-sodium broth
- 1/2 cup frozen petite green peas
- 1/3 cup grated Parmesan cheese
- 2 tablespoons chiffonade fresh basil
- 1 teaspoon lemon zest

- 1/4 cup heavy cream

- Juice of 1 lemon

- Salt and freshly ground black pepper

Instructions:

- In a medium saucepan, heat olive oil over medium-high heat. Saute diced onion until fragrant and translucent.
- Add orzo or pearl barley and toast for 2 minutes, stirring occasionally.
- Pour in the dry white wine and cook until absorbed.
- Gradually add chicken stock, stirring frequently. Bring to a simmer, lower the heat, and cover. Cook for 8 to 10 minutes until the liquid is almost absorbed, and the orzo is tender. Remove from heat.

- Stir in frozen peas, grated Parmesan, fresh basil, lemon zest, heavy cream, and lemon juice.
- Season with salt and freshly ground black pepper to taste. Serve.

Nutrition Facts (Per Serving):

- Calories: 468
- Total Fat: 17g
- Saturated Fat: 7g
- Carbohydrates: 61g
- Dietary Fiber: 14g
- Sugar: 5g
- Protein: 15g
- Cholesterol: 29mg
- Sodium: 880mg

Creamy Mushroom Risotto

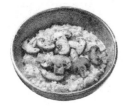

Ingredients:

- 1 tablespoon olive oil
- 12 ounces mushrooms, thinly sliced
- ¼ cup yellow onion, chopped
- 2 tablespoons salted butter
- 1 cup arborio rice
- ½ cup white wine or extra broth
- 3 cups chicken broth (divided) or mushroom broth
- ⅓ cup Parmesan cheese, freshly grated
- Fresh parsley for garnish (optional)

Instructions:

- Warm the broth in the microwave or bring it to a low simmer in a saucepan.
- In a pan over medium-high heat, add olive oil and mushrooms. Cook until mushrooms are softened (about 5 minutes). Set aside.
- Add butter and onions to a saucepan. Cook until tender (about 3-4 minutes). Stir in rice and cook until it lightly browns (about 5 minutes).
- Add wine and cook until evaporated, stirring. Add warmed broth ½ cup at a time, stirring until evaporated after each addition. This will take about 20 minutes.
- Stir in mushrooms with any juices, Parmesan cheese, and parsley. Taste and add salt & pepper as needed. Garnish with fresh herbs if desired.

Nutrition Facts (Per Serving):

- Calories: 358
- Carbohydrates: 46g
- Protein: 11g
- Fat: 13g
- Saturated Fat: 6g
- Cholesterol: 22mg
- Sodium: 831mg
- Potassium: 586mg
- Fiber: 3g
- Sugar: 3g
- Vitamin A: 247IU
- Vitamin C: 15mg
- Calcium: 109mg
- Iron: 3mg

Spaghetti Aglio e Olio

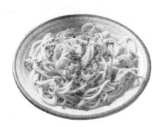

Ingredients:

- 12 ounces spaghetti
- Kosher salt
- ½ cup extra virgin olive oil
- 8 garlic cloves, thinly sliced
- ½ teaspoon red pepper flakes (optional, or more to your liking)
- ⅓ cup grated Parmesan (optional, or more to your liking)
- Chopped parsley (optional, for garnish)

Instructions:

- Bring a large pot of water to a boil. Salt the water well. Once boiling, add the pasta and cook until just before al dente. Reserve 1 ½ cups of the pasta's cooking water.
- Warm the olive oil in a large pan over medium heat. Add the garlic and stir until it's just beginning to turn golden brown.

- When the garlic has started to brown, add the red pepper flakes (if using) and toss for 30 seconds or so. Move off the heat if the pasta is not ready.
- Return to medium heat if needed. Whisk the reserved pasta water into the oil and bring to a simmer until the liquid reduces by about ⅓.
- Add the cooked pasta and stir until coated in the sauce and cooked to your liking. Turn off the heat and add Parmesan and parsley if using. Toss once more to combine.
- Allow the pasta to rest for a couple of minutes before serving. Optionally, enjoy with more Parmesan and red pepper flakes on the side.

Nutrition Facts (Per Serving):

- Calories: 399.8

- Carbohydrates: 44g
- Protein: 9.8g
- Saturated Fat: 3.6g
- Cholesterol: 4.9mg
- Sodium: 92.1mg
- Potassium: 152.9mg
- Fiber: 2g
- Sugar: 1.6g
- Vitamin A: 97.8IU
- Vitamin C: 1.3mg
- Calcium: 81.5mg
- Iron: 1mg

CHAPTER 8: SLOW-COOKED BLISS

Crockpot Chili Con Carne

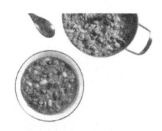

Ingredients:

- 3 lbs. extra lean ground beef
- 1 medium onion, chopped
- 1 large green pepper, chopped
- 4 garlic cloves, minced
- 1 28 oz. can tomato sauce
- 1 28 oz. can diced tomatoes, drained
- 1 10.75 oz. can tomato soup
- 2 14 oz. cans beans in tomato sauce
- 1 15 oz. can of kidney beans, rinsed

- 2 tablespoons chili powder
- 1 tablespoon dried oregano
- ½ tablespoon dried basil
- 1 teaspoon salt

Instructions:

- In a large skillet, cook ground beef for 5 minutes on medium-high. Add onion, green pepper, and garlic. Cook for an additional 5 minutes until the beef is no longer pink. Add to the crockpot.
- Add remaining ingredients and stir to combine. Cook on high for 3-4 hours or on low for 6-7 hours.
- Serve in bowls and garnish with your choice of toppings.

Suggested garnishes: Sour Cream, grated cheese, sliced green onions

Tips:

- If you prefer more spiciness, add hot sauce, cayenne pepper, or other desired spicy ingredients.
- Use any canned beans you have in your pantry, such as black beans, cannellini beans, or lentils.
- Browning the ground beef before adding it to the crockpot enhances the flavor, so don't skip this step.
- Like most stews, chili con carne tastes even better the next day, making it great for meal prep

Nutrition Facts (Per Serving):

- Calories: 464 kcal
- Carbohydrates: 46g
- Protein: 48g

- Fat: 11g
- Saturated Fat: 5g
- Cholesterol: 112mg
- Sodium: 1654mg
- Potassium: 1744mg
- Fiber: 13g
- Sugar: 12g
- Vitamin A: 1377IU
- Vitamin C: 41mg
- Calcium: 161mg
- Iron: 10mg

Moroccan Lentil Stew

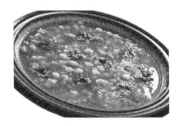

Ingredients:

- 5 cups hot water

- 2 cubes tomato bouillon with chicken flavoring
- 1 tablespoon extra-virgin olive oil
- 1 cup chopped yellow onion
- 2 large cloves garlic, minced
- 1 teaspoon dried fenugreek leaves
- 1 bay leaf
- ½ teaspoon ground cumin
- ½ teaspoon ground coriander
- ½ teaspoon ground cinnamon
- ½ teaspoon salt
- ¼ teaspoon cayenne pepper
- 1 cup lentils
- 1 cup peeled and chopped butternut squash
- 1 large carrot, chopped
- 1 celery stalk, chopped
- ½ cup chopped fresh green beans
- ¼ cup frozen peas
- 1 tablespoon chopped fresh cilantro (optional)

Instructions:

- Dissolve tomato bouillon cubes in hot water.
- Heat olive oil in a Dutch oven. Add onion, garlic, fenugreek leaves, bay leaf, cumin, coriander, cinnamon, salt, and cayenne pepper. Cook until fragrant.
- Stir in lentils, butternut squash, carrot, celery, and tomato bouillon. Bring to a boil, then simmer for 45 minutes.
- Add green beans and peas. Cook until tender. Garnish with cilantro.

Nutrition Facts (Per Serving):

- Calories: 175
- Total Fat: 3g
- Saturated Fat: 0g
- Sodium: 248mg
- Total Carbohydrate: 29g

- Dietary Fiber: 12g
- Total Sugars: 4g
- Protein: 10g
- Vitamin C: 13mg
- Calcium: 64mg
- Iron: 3mg
- Potassium: 547mg

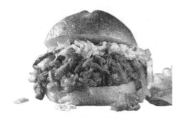

Vegan Pulled BBQ Jackfruit

Ingredients:

- 1 20 oz. can green (young) jackfruit in brine or water
- 1 tablespoon extra virgin olive oil
- ½ white onion, chopped
- 2 cloves garlic, minced

- ½ cup BBQ sauce (vegan if necessary)
- ½ cup water

Instructions:

- Drain and rinse jackfruit.
- In a stockpot, heat olive oil, and sauté onion and garlic until soft.
- Add jackfruit, BBQ sauce, and water. Cook for 5-10 minutes.
- Mash jackfruit to create a pulled meat consistency. Simmer for 15-20 minutes.
- Serve in sandwiches, tacos, or by itself.

Nutrition Facts (Per Serving):

- Calories: 131
- Total Fat: 5g
- Saturated Fat: 1g

- Sodium: 494mg
- Carbohydrates: 21g
- Fiber: 1g
- Sugar: 16g
- Protein: 1g

Printed in Great Britain
by Amazon

Book brief

1 *The Wind in the Willows* is one of the classics of children's literature.

2 The story shows Scottish writer Kenneth Grahame's love of nature that started when he was a child.

3 The story uses the adventures of four animals to teach children about what is right and wrong. It also shows how important friendship is.

4 The book quickly became popular and there are many films and plays based on the story.

5 Adults enjoy this story as much as children do because the animals have interesting human characteristics even if they still have their normal animal habits.

In this reader:

 21st Century Skills
To encourage students to connect the story to the world they live in.

 Movers
A1 level activities.

Story Notes
A brief summary of the text.

Glossary
Explanation of difficult words.

Picture Caption
A brief explanation of the picture.

Audio
These icons indicate the parts of the story that are recorded.
▶ start
■ stop

Think
To encourage students to develop their critical thinking skills.

Kenneth Grahame

The Wind
in the Willows

Retold by
Michael Lacey Freeman

Illustrated by
Andrea Rivola

Teen ELi Readers

Teen Eli Readers

The **ELI Readers** collection is a complete range of books and plays for readers of all ages, ranging from captivating contemporary stories to timeless classics. There are four series, each catering for a different age group: **First ELI Readers, Young ELI Readers, Teen ELI Readers** and **Young Adult ELI Readers**. The books are carefully edited and beautifully illustrated to capture the essence of the stories and plots. The readers are supplemented with 'Focus on' texts packed with background cultural information about the writers and their lives and times.

The Wind in the Willows
by Kenneth Grahame
Adaptation and activities by
Michael Lacey Freeman
Language Level Consultants
Lisa Suett and Silvana Sardi
Illustrations by **Andrea Rivola**

ELI Readers
Founder and Series Editors
Paola Accattoli, Grazia Ancillani, Daniele Garbuglia (Art Director)

Graphic Design
**Andersen
the Premedia Company**

Production Manager
Francesco Capitano

Photo credits
Shutterstock

New edition: **2021**
First edition: **2019**

© **ELI s.r.l.**
P.O. Box 6
62019 Recanati (MC)
Italy
T +39 071750701
F +39 071977851
info@elionline.com
www.elionline.com

Typeset in 12 / 17 pt
Fulmar designed by Leo Philp

Printed in Italy by
**Tecnostampa - Pigini Group
Printing Division
Loreto - Trevi (Italia) -
ERT 129.10
ISBN 978-88-536-3191-6**

Contents

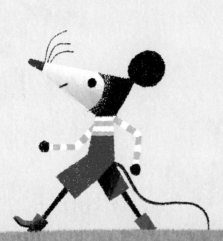

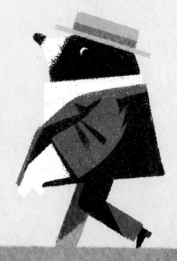

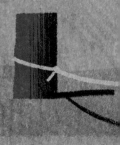

Rat

*He loves the river and is always
ready to help his friends.*

Mole

*He doesn't know much about the
world but he likes adventures.*

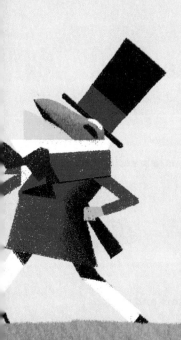

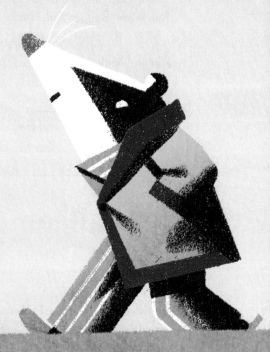

Toad

He's rich, he loves talking about himself, and he doesn't usually listen to his friends.

Badger

He's very clever and tells Toad to stop doing silly things.

Reading and Writing MOVERS

1 Choose the correct word for each sentence.

The Wind in the Willows is ___*a*___ story about four friends:
Rat, Mole, Badger and Toady.

a	one	an

1 Rat and Mole _____ by the river.

lives	live	doesn't live

2 Badger lives _____ the Wild Wood and Toad lives in
a big house called Toad Hall.

on	to	in

3 The story _____ about how friends help each other.

is	am	are

4 Toad does a _____ of silly things.

lot	many	much

Reading

**2 Read the descriptions of the main characters and match
them with the pictures on pages 6 & 7.**

1 The Mole   He wants to see the world.
2 The Rat   He's a good friend.
3 The Toad   He likes an exciting life.
4 The Badger   He knows a lot of things and tries to help his friends.

Writing

**3 The story is called, *The Wind in the Willows*. A willow is a tree.
What other things from nature do you think are in the story?**

Trees	Wind	

21st
Century
Skills

Chapter 1

My World

▶2 'It's Spring outside,' thought Mole[1]. 'The flowers, the grass, the sun, the sweet music of the birds. I really want to see and hear it all. But first I have to clean my house. It's very dirty.'

Mole looked around his dark house. 'I have to clean the kitchen, and the bedroom, and the bathroom and ... and.' But Mole couldn't finish his sentence.

He couldn't stop thinking of...

Outside!

Up there!

He thought of his favourite flowers, the green grass, the gentle[2] wind and the hot sun and said,

'It's no good. I have to go out. I have to go...

Up!

Up!

Up!'

So he left his house, and soon he was out of his dark home, and into the light of the spring.

Mole was so happy that he started running. He felt the grass under his feet, and the air[3] against

---

[1] **mole**
[2] **gentle** not strong
[3] **air** wind

his face. He didn't stop. He couldn't stop. Soon he arrived at the other side of the field.

'This is life!' said Mole.

Then Mole stopped. He could see the river, and he looked at the water. 'The sun is dancing on the water!' he said to himself.

He looked and looked. He couldn't move! It was so beautiful!

'The river is talking to me!' he thought.

Then Mole listened again. It wasn't the river that talked, it was something else. It was an animal on the other side of the river.

'Hello!' it said.

Mole looked at the animal. It had a brown face, small ears and thick hair.

It was Rat!

'Hello, Rat!' said Mole.

'Hi, Mole! Come here and speak to me.'

'I don't want to talk now,' said Mole. There were more important things to do than talking.

But when Rat got into a little boat to cross the river, Mole talked a little more, this time to himself.

'Oh! I love boats,' he said.

'Get in!' said Rat.

Mole got in the boat. At first he was worried. He couldn't swim. Was it safe?

But soon Mole was in the middle of the river, moving along very slowly, in a little boat made for two.

'This is so relaxing¹' said Mole. 'My first time in a boat. I'm so excited.'

'Really,' said Rat. 'Your first time?'

'Yes, and it's really nice,' replied Mole.

'Nice!' said the Rat. 'It's more than nice. It's the ONLY thing to do. The great thing about boats is that it's fun all the time. You don't have to go anywhere. Let's go out for the day.'

'Where?' asked Mole.

'Nowhere,' said Rat.

'Let's go nowhere now!' said Mole.

So that's where they went. It was nice for Mole to go nowhere. 'I always know where I'm going. It's nice to not know, just for one day.'

'So, this is a river!' said Mole to his new friend.

'It's not a river. It's THE river!' replied Rat. 'It's my world. It's everything. Winter, or summer, spring or autumn.

'What's that over there?' asked Mole, pointing to his left.

Mole meets a new friend, Rat, and they go down the river in a boat. Mole loves it. The river is new for Mole but Rat knows the river very well and loves it. It's his world.

¹ **relaxing** when something stops you feeling worried

11

'Oh, that's The Wild Wood. I don't go there.'

'Why?'

'It's a strange[1] and dangerous place. It's not safe.'

'If you walk to the end of the woods, what can you see?' asked Mole.

'After the woods there's the rest of the world. I don't want to go there and I don't want to see it. This is enough[2] for me,' said Rat looking at the river.

After saying this, the two friends stopped to have lunch. They left the boat and had a picnic on the grass.

Mole was so happy, and so hungry. There was cold chicken and sandwiches, salad and orange juice. The two friends were very hungry, and soon they finished everything.

After the picnic, Rat and Mole got into the boat again. The afternoon sun was low[3] in the sky, and the two friends didn't talk very much.

But then Mole wanted to look at The Wild Wood again. 'Look!' he said, standing up in the boat.

Standing up in a boat isn't very easy. The boat moved, Rat moved, Mole moved. And suddenly[4],

SPLASH!

Rat doesn't like The Wild Wood and he doesn't want to know about the rest of the world. All he needs is the river.

Think

Who likes doing new things more, Mole or Rat?

[1] **strange** not something you usually see or do
[2] **enough** all you need
[3] **low** when the sun goes down, it's low in the sky
[4] **suddenly** when something happens quickly and you're surprised

Rat and Mole are having fun going down the river in Rat's boat.

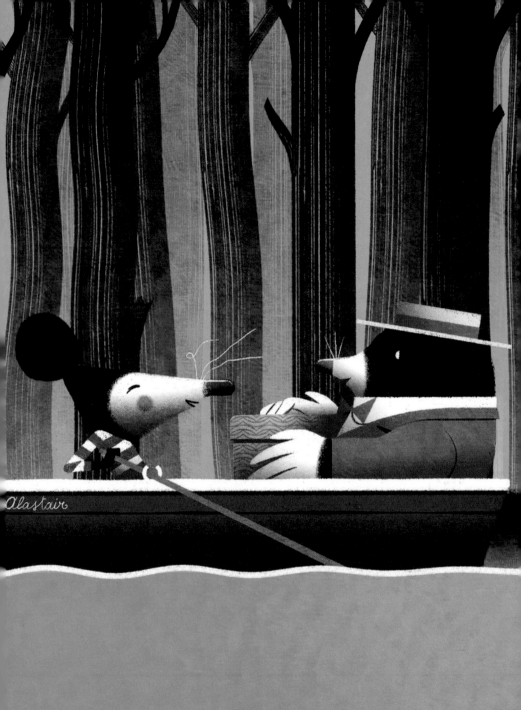

Rat and Mole were in the river, and the river was very, very cold.

'Help! Help!' cried Mole. He was frightened. But soon he felt someone pulling him to the bank[1]. It was Rat. He was laughing.

Mole stands up in the boat to see The Wild Wood and the two friends fall into the river. Mole can't swim but Rat helps him. Rat isn't angry with Mole.

When they were on the bank, Rat said, 'Now my friend, rest[2] for a few minutes. I need to go back into the river to get our boat.'

'I'm so sorry,' said Mole.

'That's all right,' said Rat. 'I'm in the water all the time. Don't worry.'

Rat was so kind[3]!

'I have to go home now. It's late,' said Mole when they were ready to get back in the boat.

'Home!' said Rat. 'No, you aren't going home. You're coming home with me. We have many adventures[4] in front of us with our boat. You can't go home now.'

That's why at the end of the day, Mole went home with Rat. That evening Rat made a fire[5] to get warm, and told the Mole stories until tea time.

They were very interesting[6] stories, all about

---

[1] **bank** the side of the river
[2] **rest** sit quietly
[3] **kind** nice, good
[4] **adventure** something exciting you do

[5] **fire**
[6] **interesting** something that you want to listen to, watch or read about

life in the water, and boats and birds, and many other animals. He often told stories about a friend called, Toad[1]. He seemed to be a very interesting animal indeed.

'Toad is very friendly, and very rich[2]. He's always happy to see people. He's not very clever, and sometimes he's like a little child, but he has a good heart.'

Spring became summer, and Mole spent all of his time with Rat. He didn't go back to his dark home. He learnt to swim, and began to love the water and life on the river more and more every day.

Then, one summer day, Mole decided[3] to ask Rat something.

'Can you take me to see Toad?' I really want to meet him.

'Certainly[4],' said Rat. 'Let's get the boat and go there now.'

The journey[5] was very short, and soon they saw a big white house with a beautiful garden.

'There's Toad Hall!' said Rat. 'Let's get out of the boat.'

Mole stays with Rat and learns to swim and love the water. One day they visit Rat's rich friend, Toad, who lives in a big house.

[1] **toad**
[2] **rich** someone who has a lot of money
[3] **decide** to think about something and then do it
[4] **certainly** of course
[5] **journey** the time you travel on a bus, train or boat

The two friends walked across the garden, and soon they saw Toad, sitting on a chair, and looking at a large map.

'Hooray!' said Toad when he saw Rat and Mole. 'Nice to see you! I'm really happy you're here. You have to help me. It's something really important. Come with me!'

And so Mole and Rat followed[1] Toad into a garage[2], where they saw a cart[3]. The cart was yellow and it even had yellow wheels[4].

'There you are!' said Toad. 'There's real life for you. Better than the river. The open road! We can see villages, towns and cities. We leave this afternoon. Everything is ready.'

Mole was very excited, and wanted to look inside the cart. The inside of the cart looked very comfortable[5]. There was a place to sleep and cook. And Mole was even more excited when he saw the biscuits and the jam[6].

But Rat wasn't so sure[7]. 'Sorry,' he said slowly. 'Did you say the words 'We' and 'Leave' and 'This Afternoon'?' ■

Toad is happy to see Rat and Mole and wants to take them on a trip in his cart. Mole is excited about this idea but Rat isn't very happy about it.

❯

Mole, Toad and Rat are sitting aroun the fire havir something to eat and the cart and hors are behind Toad. Toad wants to go o a trip with hi friends in the cart.

---

[1] **follow** to walk behind someone
[2] **garage** where people put their car at home
[3] **cart** see picture on page 17
[4] **wheel** 🛞
[5] **comfortable** nice and warm
[6] **jam**
[7] **sure** happy about something

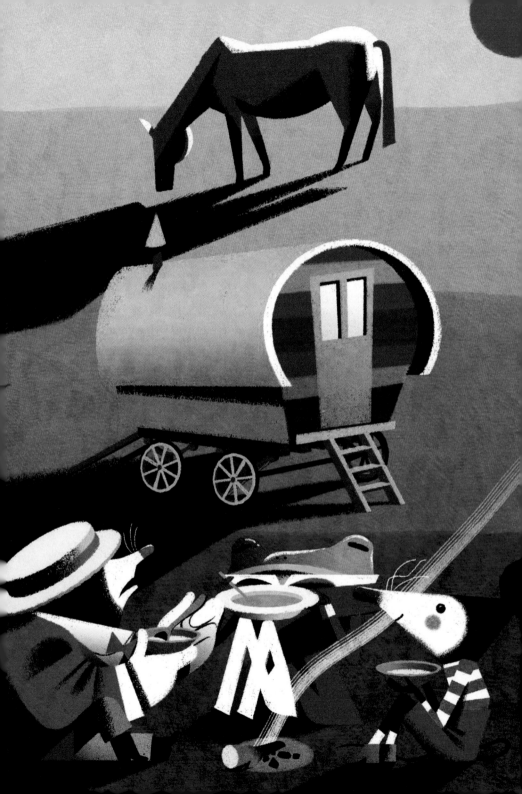

Speaking and Writing

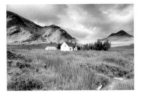 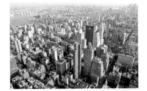

 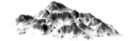 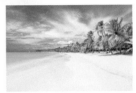

1 In Chapter 1 Toad wants to go on a trip with Mole and Rat. Discuss these questions with a partner and write your answers.

1 Why do you think Mole likes Toad's idea more than Rat?

2 What kind of new things do you like doing?

3 Do you prefer visiting a place in the countryside or a big city? Why?

4 Do you prefer the beach or the mountains? Why?

5 Do you think it's important to travel and see new places? Why / Why not?

6 Which countries would you like to visit? Why?

Reading Comprehension

2 Number these sentences in the order that they happen in Chapter 1.

a ☐ Rat and Mole go on a boat.

b ☐ Rat and Mole go to Rat's house.

c ☐ Rat and Mole are in the water.

d ☐ Rat and Mole visit Toad.

e ☑ Mole meets Rat.

f ☐ Rat and Mole have a picnic.

Reading and Writing MOVERS

3 Choose the correct word(s) for each sentence.

Mole's house is very ___dirty___ .

> clean ~~dirty~~ in a tree

1 It's _____ outside.

> cold   rainy   warm

2 Rat has got _____ .

> big ears   a white face   thick hair

3 Rat _____ the river

> likes   don't like   like

4 Rat and Mole have a picnic on the _____ .

> boat   grass   river

5 Mole wants _____ Toad.

> meet   to meet   meeting

Before-reading Activities

Speaking

4 The next chapter is called 'The Wild Wood'. Why do you think that this is the title?

Listening

▶ 3 **5 Look at the last words of Chapter 1 again.**
'Did you say the words 'We' and 'Leave' and 'This Afternoon'?'
Did Rat, Mole and Toad leave?
Listen to the first part of Chapter 2 to hear the answer.

Chapter 2

The Wild Wood

▶ 3 Mole opened his eyes and looked out of the cart. It was a beautiful morning.

'Morning, Mole,' said Rat, who was awake too. 'Look at Toad, he's still sleeping!'

Mole and Rat went outside to have some breakfast. Toad looked so happy in his sleep. They didn't want to wake him.

'I'm excited about today,' said Mole. 'Are we going nowhere again?'

Rat didn't answer his friend. He wanted to go somewhere. He wanted to go back to his river.

Mole understood. 'Do you want to go back?'

'No, it's alright,' said Rat. 'I think Toad is getting bored¹ of this.'

Rat was right.

Rat and Mole waited for hours for Toad to wake up, and when he did, they began the day's journey. It was a sunny day, and they met many birds, and rabbits, and other friendly animals. In the afternoon they stopped for lunch. ■

¹ **get bored of** when you feel unhappy because something isn't interesting

20

▶4　Mole picked up a chicken sandwich, but before he could eat he heard a noise,

Vroooooommmmm!

It was a car, and it went past them so quickly. The noise frightened the horse, the cart began to move from one side of the road to the other, and then,

CRASH!

The yellow cart was on the ground, and so were Rat, Mole and Toad.

Rat was very angry. 'Some people are so stupid[1],' he said loudly. But then Rat looked at Toad. He was in the middle of the road, sitting there and looking at the car, which was now very far away.

'Are you okay?' asked Mole. 'Toad, are you alright?'

But all Toad could say was, 'The Car! The REAL way to travel. The ONLY way to travel.'

'Stop it!' said Rat. 'Help us with the cart.'

'No more carts,' said Toad. 'The Car!!!!!!'

'Toad doesn't want to move.' said Mole.

'Let's leave him,' said Rat. 'Now Toad has a

Rat and Mole like travelling in the cart but Toad doesn't like it anymore. He wants to travel by car!

---

[1] **stupid** someone stupid does things without thinking

21

new interest. Cars. There's nothing we can do.

I know him.'

Rat and Mole left Toad, sitting there in the road, and they went back to the river they loved so much.

Mole wants to meet Badger who lives in the Wild Wood. It's winter and Rat sleeps a lot so Mole decides to go on his own to visit Badger.

The next day, Toad bought a large[1] and very expensive[2] car!

After meeting Toad, Mole really wanted to meet another friend of Rat: Badger[3]. Everybody talked about him. But Badger was difficult to find.

Every time Mole asked about meeting Badger, Rat said. 'We can go soon.'

But soon never arrived. Winter arrived instead[4]. When it started to get cold, Rat slept a lot, so one day, Mole decided to go on his own[5] to find the Badger. The only problem was that he lived in the Wild Wood!

It was cold when Mole went out and there were so many trees.

Mole started to get frightened. He could hear some strange noises.

Fweeeeeeeeee!

[1] **large** big
[2] **expensive** you need a lot of money to buy something expensive
[3] **badger**
[4] **instead** in place of another thing
[5] **on his own** only him

Where did the noise come from? Was it the leaves falling? Or was it the wind?

Then he heard something moving to his right. Wooooossssh!

It was too much. It was too frightening[1]. Mole started to run. He ran and ran until he could run no more. By now he was far from his home, in the middle of the woods.

He was tired; so tired!

So he stopped next to a big tree.

'Now I know why this place is called The Wild Wood,' he thought before he fell asleep.

Rat went into the woods to look for his friend. The sun was almost down. He looked left and right.

'Mole! Mole! Where are you? It's me! It's Rat!'

After about an hour, Rat heard someone crying. It was Mole. Rat found him by the tree.

'Oh, Rat! Thank goodness[2] you're here. I'm so frightened.'

'Don't worry,' said Rat. 'I told you not to go out in the Wild Wood, especially alone[3].'

Mole is very frightened in the Wild Wood, but his friend, Rat finds him. They sleep there and when they wake up next morning, everything is white.

[1] **frightening** scary
[2] **Thank goodness!** phew! great!
[3] **alone** only you, no other people

Both Rat and Mole were so tired, and they fell asleep under the tree. When the two friends finally woke up, they wanted to go home. But when they opened their eyes and looked at the trees, they saw that they were white!

'It's snowing,' said Rat. 'Quickly, we have to go now before everything gets white.'

The woods looked very different now. Rat tried to remember the way home, but it was difficult.

After an hour, they were still lost. Home was still so far away!

'We need to find a hole[1]; somewhere we can stay dry and rest,' said Rat to Mole. But Mole wasn't there! Rat looked around. He couldn't see Mole, but he could hear him.

Mole falls down a hole and Rat goes to help him. Then they see a green door. It's Badger's house!

'Help me!' said Mole. 'I'm in a hole!'

'I'm coming,' said Rat. 'Wait there!'

Rat went down the hole to help his friend.

'Here I am,' said Rat. 'But wait! I know this hole! Look!'

The two friends looked and saw a green door in front of them. They knocked[2] on the door and waited for what seemed to be a very long time before the door opened, just a little.

❯

When Rat and Mole wake up in Wild Wood everything white and th don't know how to get home.

---

[1] **hole**
[2] **knock** hit the door with your hand

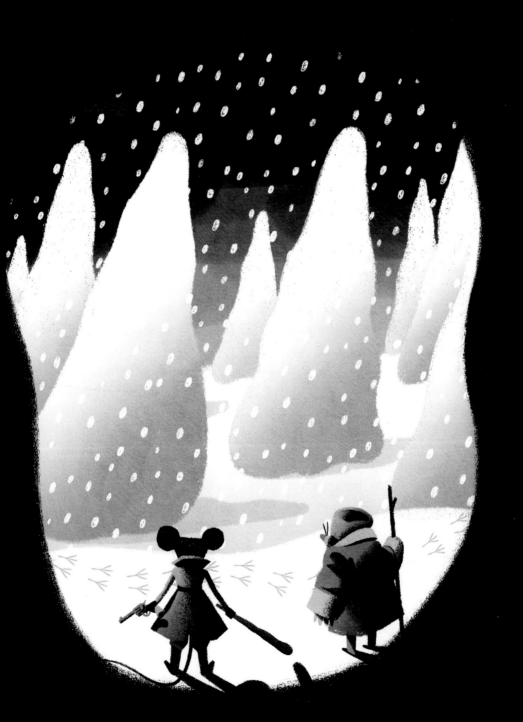

Kenneth Grahame

'Who is it?' said Badger.

'Oh, Badger,' said Rat. 'Let us in please!'

'Oh, it's you, Rat!' said Badger. 'Come in.'

Rat and Mole followed Badger into the house, and soon they were in a very large kitchen that had a great big fire.

Suddenly the Wild Wood seemed so far away, like a bad dream. Soon the three animals were sitting around a table with all kinds of delicious[1] food in front of them.

'What luck[2]!' said Rat. 'We're so happy that we saw your door!'

While they ate, the three animals started to talk about Toad. 'How is Toad?' asked Badger.

'Pretty bad[3],' said Rat. 'He can't drive properly[4], and he keeps having[5] accidents[6].'

'When summer comes, we can visit him' said Badger. 'But now, it's time for bed.'

'What an adventure!' said Rat.

'Yes,' said Mole. 'I don't know what can happen next.' ◉

Rat tells Badger that Toad isn't good at driving. Badger says they can visit him in summer.

❯

Rat and Mo are happy n in Badger's house. The are lots of nice things to eat and i safe here, n like the Wi Wood abov them.

Think

Can you think of any new adventures for Badger, Mole and Rat?

[1] **delicious** very good (for food)
[2] **luck** something good
[3] **pretty bad** not very good
[4] **properly** correctly
[5] **keep having** have again and again
[6] **accident** what happens to the cart in chapter 1

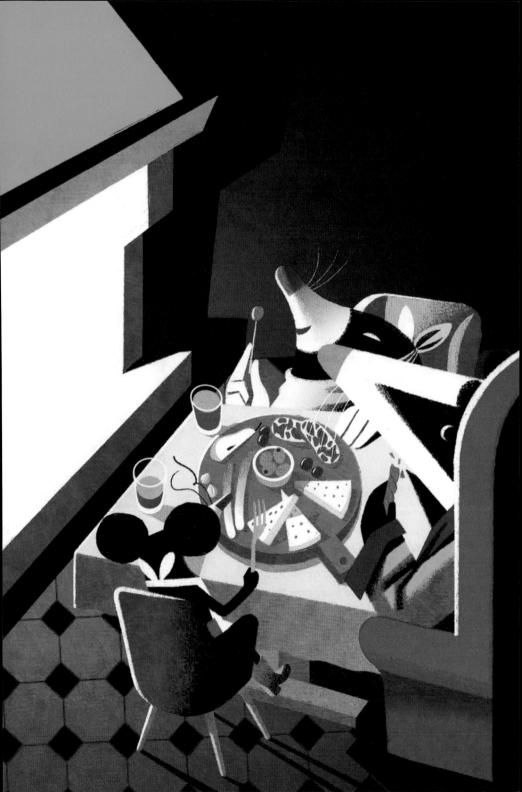

Reading Comprehension

1 Read the sentences and tick 3 the ones you think are true.

☑ Mole woke up early.
1 ☐ Rat invites Mole to go back to the river.
2 ☐ Toad doesn't like the car.
3 ☐ Mole wants to meet Badger.
4 ☐ Rat goes to the Wild Wood with Badger.
5 ☐ There's a lot of light in the Wild Wood.
6 ☐ Rat and Mole get lost in the Wild Wood.

Reading and Writing MOVERS

2 Look at the picture on page 27. Complete the sentences and answer the questions.

Rat and Mole are with ___*Badger*___ .
1 What colour is the fork in Rat's hand?
_____
2 Rat is sitting opposite _____ .
3 How many glasses are there on the table?
_____
4 What are the friends doing?
_____

3 Read the sentences and decide who they describe.

He sometimes gets frightened.   ___*Mole*___
1 He likes to learn new things.   _____
2 He likes his normal life.   _____
3 He gets excited very quickly.   _____
4 He knows Toad very well.   _____
5 He's very rich.   _____
6 People don't see him very often.   _____

28

Speaking

4 Play this game with a partner. Say a sentence about someone you both know, but don't say the name of the person.
Your partner has to tell you the person's name.
You can use some of the sentences in exercise 3 to help you.

> *Example:*
> *A: He loves dogs.*
> *B: Are you talking about Brian?*
> *A: No, sorry. He can ride a bike too.*
> *B: James?*
> *A: Yes, that's right!*

21st Century Skills

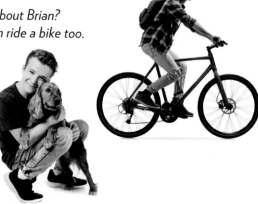

Before-reading Activities

Speaking

5 The next chapter is called, 'Home'. Which home do you think it is about? Why?

a ☐ Rat's home
b ☐ Badger's home
c ☐ Mole's home

Listening

▶ 6 **6** Listen to track 6. Do Rat and Mole:

a ☐ leave Badger?
b ☐ stay with Badger?

Chapter 3

Home

▶ 5 It was breakfast-time at Badger's house, and Mole wanted to know more about The Wild Wood.

'How old is the Wild Wood?' asked Mole.

'Well, a long time ago, before the trees, before the Wild Wood, there was a city – a city of people.'

'Really? What happened to those people?' asked Mole.

'Nobody knows,' said Badger. 'People come and go, but we animals remain[1]. There were badgers before people, and there will be badgers after people. When the people left, the wood grew. Maybe people will come back again one day. But for now, the Wild Wood is ours.' ■

▶ 6 Rat was happy that the Wild Wood belonged[2] to the animals but, after breakfast he wanted to leave. Rat wanted to go home. 'I don't want to spend another night in the Wild Wood,' he said.

Badger took them to the door, and said goodbye.

Badger says that before there was a city with people in the Wild Wood but now there are only animals. Rat wants to go home so Mole leaves with him.

[1] **remain** stay
[2] **belong** when something is yours it belongs to you

In the light of day, even with the snow, it was easy to find the road. Very soon Rat and Mole were out of the Wild Wood. They saw the river in front of them – in the distance[1]. Their river! ◉

7   When they arrived at the field they were very near to Rat's home! But then Mole lifted[2] his nose up into the air. There was something - something he knew really well. A smell[3]. What was that smell?

Home! Mole's home!

His old house! He was near! His house was calling to him.

'Rat!' he called. 'Rat!'

But Rat couldn't hear. Rat was walking home and thinking of his dinner.

'Rat,' called Mole again. 'It's my home, my old house. Come back! Please come back!'

But Rat was too far away now. He couldn't hear what his friend was saying.

Mole had to think. It was hard. He looked towards his house, and to Rat's house. 'What can I do?' he thought. 'I have to follow Rat. I can't leave him.' So Mole ran to his friend.

---

[1] **in the distance** not near
[2] **lift** put up
[3] **smell** you do this with your nose

While they walked, Mole was silent[1]. At first, Rat thought that Mole was tired,

'We're nearly home.'

'Home?' said Mole. Where was home?

Mole sat by a tree and tried to rest, but he could not stop himself, and started to cry.

'What is it my friend?' asked Rat.

'It's not like your warm, comfortable house, or Toad's or Badger's but it's my own little home – and I need it. It called to me and I wanted it. I just want to take one look at it.'

Rat waited for his friend to stop crying and then he said, 'Well, let's go.'

'Where?' asked Mole.

'To find your house, my friend. Take my arm.'

They didn't have to walk very far before Mole's nose started to move up and down.

'I smell something,' he said.

Mole walked, and Rat followed. They were in the field, when suddenly Mole disappeared[2]. Rat followed and saw a little hole. And then Rat went

Down! Down! Down!

Until he saw it. Mole's little front door.

Mole likes adventures but he wants to go home too, so Rat goes with him.

---

[1] **silent** when you don't say anything
[2] **to disappear** to not be there anymore.

When Rat opened the door, he saw Mole's face! Mole was home!

But Mole's face wasn't happy exactly[1].

'Oh Rat! Why did I bring you to this cold, dirty place?'

'What a lovely house!' cried Rat. 'Everything is in its place. We can clean it a bit. Let's do it!' Mole got up and started cleaning with Rat.

After cleaning, Mole sat down in silence and fell asleep thinking that it was quite good to have a place called home. It was good to know that he could come back to it when he needed it.

It was early summer. It was time to take out the boat. Rat and Mole were getting ready when they heard a knock at the door.

Mole went to the door, and was very surprised to see Badger!

Badger looked very worried indeed[2] when he said,

'We have to see Toad now that the weather is fine. I think he needs our help. He's waiting for a new car to arrive. We must go and see him, and try to stop him from driving.

Rat, Mole and Badger are worried about Toad who is waiting for a new car to arrive, so they go to Toad Hall.

---

[1] **not exactly** not at all
[2] **indeed** really

That's why, the next day, they went to Toad Hall.

When Rat, Mole and Badger went through the gate[1] they saw something big, and red, and new.

'Look,' said Mole. 'It's too late. Toad has got his new car.'

When they knocked on the door, Toad opened it with a big smile on his face. 'Hello! Come in!' he cried. 'We can go somewhere in my new, my new, new ...'

But Toad stopped speaking because he noticed[2] the expression[3] on the faces of his friends.

'Toad, can I speak to you alone for five minutes?' asked Badger.

'Yes, of course,' said Toad.

Toad and Badger went into the living room, and Badger began to speak.

'They can put you in prison[4] for driving so fast. Don't get in a car again!'

The two animals spoke for an hour. Rat and Mole tried to listen outside the door, but they couldn't hear anything.

When the door opened, Toad and Badger came out. Toad looked very quiet.

[1] **gate**
[2] **notice** see
[3] **expression** how you look
[4] **prison** look at the picture on page 37. Toad is in this place.

'Sit down Toad,' said Badger.

Toad sat down while Badger started to tell Rat and Mole everything.

'My friends, I want to tell you that Toad understands now that it's better to stop using the car.'

'That's good news[1]!' said Mole.

'Yes, very good,' said Rat.

But while Rat spoke he noticed a smile on Toad's face.

'No, I'm NOT sorry,' said Toad suddenly. 'It isn't stupid to drive a car. It's wonderful[2].'

'But, but, but,' said Badger. 'In the living room you said something different.'

'You're right, Badger. I said "sorry" in the living room. I had to say "sorry" and "of course" in the living room with you because you're so clever. But I didn't mean it. I just can't say goodbye to my new red car. It's so fast!'

'Faster! Faster!' shouted Toad.

The next day Toad was in his new car. 'It's so fast,' he thought. 'But it can go faster and faster.'

Soon, Toad forgot everything. He forgot that he

Toad's friends try to tell him to stop driving so fast but he doesn't listen to them.

---

[1] **news** something new you hear or read about
[2] **wonderful** really good

was Toad of Toad Hall. He forgot what his friends said to him about driving carefully. It was just him and his car. His new red car.

Toad's smile got bigger and bigger, and his car went faster and faster.

Vroooooooommmmmmmmmmmm!!

'Badger doesn't understand,' thought Toad. 'He doesn't know how wonderful it is to have the wind against your face, to be fast, to be,

CRASH!

It was too late. Toad's car didn't look new anymore. It was in the river and Toad's smile disappeared into the river too.

Some men came. They carried Toad out of the river and took him to a big castle[1]. In the castle, there was a room; a dark and dirty room. The men took him to this room, and left him there, alone.

He was in prison.

'Why me?' Toad said to himself. 'I just wanted to have some fun. Now I'm all alone in this cold and dark place.'

Toad forgets what his friends said and drives so fast that he has a crash and the car goes into the river. Now he's in prison and very sad.

Toad is sad now becaus he's in priso for driving fast.

Think

What do you think of Toad?

[1] castle

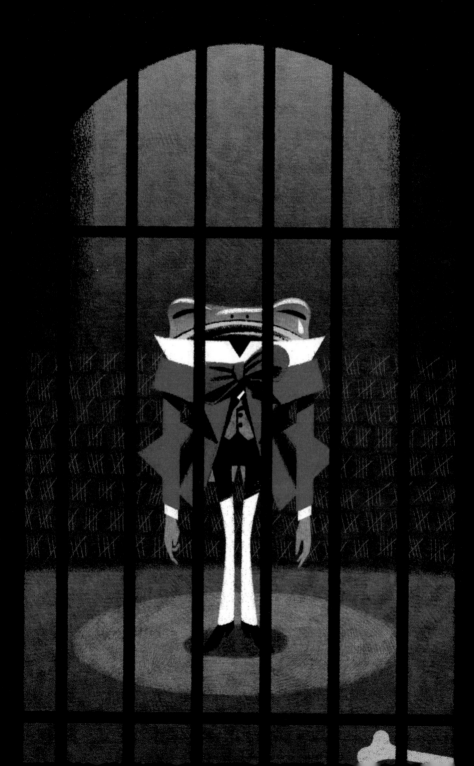

Reading and Writing   MOVERS

1 Choose the correct word for each sentence.

There ___was___ a city in the Wild Wood before the trees.

were   ~~was~~   is

1 Rat didn't want to spend _____ night in the Wild Wood.

another   more   other

2 Mole started to _____ because he was sad and wanted to go home.

laugh   cry   smile

3 Toad is waiting for a new _____.

bike   boat   car

4 Badger spoke _____ Toad about driving too fast.

for   to   at

5 Toad _____ listen to his friends.

doesn't   isn't   don't

Reading Comprehension

2 Look at the sentences and fill in the gaps with the correct word.

Rat was h _appy_ that the W _ild_ Wood belonged to the animals.

1 Rat's home was w _____ and comfortable.

2 Mole lifted his n _____ up into the air. There was something - something he knew really well.

3 'Let's find your h _____ my friend,' said Rat.

4 'What a l _____ home,' said Rat.

Vocabulary

③ Look at these words and circle the odd one out.

boat, car, cart, (wheel)

1 breakfast, dinner, lunch, sandwich
2 bed, field, river wood
3 city, house, town, village
4 bedroom, garden, kitchen, living room
5 hear, like, see, smell
6 hour, minute, month, second

Speaking

21st
Century
Skills

④ Answer these questions then show them to your partner and see if your answers are the same.

1 In the story, Mole wants to go home. How important is it to have a place you can call 'home'? Why?
2 Badger tries to tell Toad to stop driving fast. If one of your friends is doing something wrong, do you tell him /her to stop? Why / Why not?
3 Toad doesn't listen to his friends. Do you usually listen to what your friends say? Why / Why not?
4 If you have a problem, who do you talk to about it? Why?

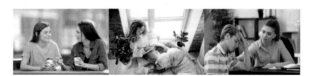

Before-reading Activity

Listening

▶ 8 **⑤ Listen to the first part of Chapter 4. Where are Rat and Mole?**

a ☐ At Toad's house.
b ☐ By the river.
c ☐ At the railway station.

Chapter 4

Run Toad, Run!

8 While[1] Toad was in prison, Rat and Mole were by the river, listening to the wind.

'Oh, Mole! The beauty of it all[2],' said Rat. 'The music of the river. It's calling us.'

Rat and Mole were happy and at peace[3]. ◼

9 But, in his small, and dark prison, Toad had no peace. 'This is the end of everything. At least, it's the end of me!' he thought. 'How can I be here? I'm an important toad. Everybody loves me.'

Toad spent four or five weeks like this, feeling sorry for himself. He thought of his comfortable bed at home, his favourite armchair, his garden. All of the things he loved were far away.

He didn't see Rat or Mole or Badger at this time. There was only one man he saw every day. He worked at the prison, and he wasn't interested in conversation. This man had a daughter, and one day she came to visit Toad.

It was nice for Toad to see someone smiling. 'Hello, Toad,' said the girl, 'would you like to talk to me?'

Toad is very sad in prison. He wants his home and his friends. Then the prison worker's daughter starts to visit him. Toad is happier because now he can talk about himself.

[1] **while** at the same time as
[2] **The beauty of it all** everything is beautiful
[3] **at peace** quiet, not angry or worried

Now one thing you must know about Toad is that he liked talking. Once he started he couldn't stop. He talked and talked – about himself, about how important he was, and how rich and clever he was. And the girl listened.

The next day, the girl came to see him with some food.

'I want you to eat,' said the girl. 'Father says you're not eating anything. That's not good for a toad'. She sat with him while he ate.

While Toad ate he talked about nice things - about green fields, the sun and wind and his garden.

Toad was happy, doing his favourite thing – talking about himself. He talked about his fish, his horses, his boat, and about the big dinner table in the dining room where he invited all his friends, and about how he sang songs and told stories.

After many hours, the girl said goodnight. Toad was happy. At last he had someone to talk to. Toad and the young girl had many interesting talks after that and the days went past a little bit more easily.

The girl felt very sorry for Toad. 'It's sad that he's in prison for doing such a little thing,' she thought.

Toad was not surprised that the girl liked him.

'Of course she likes me,' he thought. 'I'm so clever and I always say interesting things.'

One day, the girl came and gave him some clothes.

'Why do I need these clothes?' asked Toad. 'They're the clothes of a woman!'

'Wear these and people will think you're a woman. Then you can get out of this prison. You can walk out. Nobody will know that you're Toad.'

'You're a good, kind and clever girl. Thank you so much.'

The next evening, Toad put put the clothes on.

When he was ready the girl stood back and said, 'Well, you look just like an old lady[1], hahaha!'

Toad wasn't happy with what the girl said. He was Toad, and not an old lady, but now wasn't the time to say anything. Now he had to get out of prison. Toad followed the girl out of that dark room. Everybody he met inside the castle said, 'Hello, Madam!' Nobody

The girl wants to help Toad run away from prison. She brings him some clothes and when Toad puts them on he looks like and old lady. Now nobody can see it's Toad and he can run away.

[1] **lady** woman

thought he was Toad. Every person he met smiled at him and said 'Hello'.

After what seemed like forever he was in front of the gate. When he opened the gate he knew that he was free[1].

Toad thanked the girl and walked quickly into town, not knowing what to do next. As he walked along he saw some red and green lights in the distance, and he heard a sound[2] that he knew.

'Oh, what luck!' he said. 'It's a train. There's a railway station[3] nearby.' Toad made his way[4] to the station, looked at the timetable[5] and found a train that was going near his home in half an hour.

'More luck!' he said to himself and he went off to buy his ticket.

But then he remembered. Where was his money? It was in the pocket[6] of his coat! But his coat was in the prison. He had no money. He was wearing a poor woman's clothes now, not the clothes of a rich toad.

---

[1] **free** not in prison
[2] **sound** noise
[3] **railway station** train station
[4] **make (his) way** walk, go to
[5] **timetable** where you can see the train times
[6] **pocket** →

Toad walked up and down on the platform[1], where the train was waiting. 'Soon the police[2] will know I'm not there, and they will take me back to prison,' he thought. Then Toad looked at the train.

Toad runs away from prison and goes to the train station. He hasn't got any money to buy a train ticket but the kind driver says he can sit next to him, because he thinks Toad is a poor old woman.

'I can jump on and hide somewhere,' thought Toad.

Then Toad saw the driver, and he had another idea. 'Please, Mister,' said Toad, 'I'm a poor woman, and have no money, please help me'.

The driver was a kind man and so he said. 'Okay, get on. You can sit near me.'

'When I get home,' thought Toad. 'I will send this kind driver some money so he can buy some new shirts, and clothes for his family.'

The train left, and Toad looked out of the window. He could see trees and fields, horses and cows. Every minute took him nearer and nearer to Toad Hall, and his friends, and money and a nice bed to sleep in. Toad began to think about what he wanted for dinner when he heard the driver say.

[1] **platform** where you stand and wait to get on a train
[2] **police**

'That's strange, this train is the last one today. But I can see another train coming behind us'. Instantly[1], Toad knew which train it was. It was a train, full of[2] people looking for him.

Toad looked up at the moon in the sky. The moon looked free, but he didn't feel free. He could hear the train now.

'What can I do?' thought Toad.

Then Toad could not only hear the train. He put his head out of the window, and he could see the train too. 'I can see angry people,' he thought. 'I can see policemen!'

'Please help me!' said Toad to the kind driver. 'I'm not an old woman. I'm Mr. Toad. I got out of prison and those people want to take me back and make me live on bread and water and sleep on the cold floor. But I only drove a car a little too fast. Please help me!'

'You're a very bad Toad,' said the driver. 'But I don't like seeing you so sad. Don't worry, Toad. I've got a good idea.'

[1] **instantly** at that moment
[2] **full of** with a lot of

With the driver's help, Toad jumps off the train as it comes out of the tunnel and runs away from the police who are on the train behind them. That night he sleeps in the wood.

The driver made the train go faster and faster. 'There's only one thing you can do,' he said. 'We're going into a tunnel[1] now. When we come out there is a wood. When we see the wood I will slow down as much as I can so that you can jump and hide in the wood. Be ready to jump when I tell you.'

The train went faster and faster and into the tunnel. Then the driver slowed down. Toad got ready to jump...

'Now, jump!' shouted the driver.

Toad jumped.

He felt the grass under his feet and ran into the woods.

Looking from behind a tree, he saw the other train and heard people shouting - Stop! Stop! Stop!'

Toad laughed to himself. 'I am so clever.'

But soon he stopped laughing. It was late. It was dark. He was cold and hungry. Toad stayed there behind the tree. The wood seemed so unfriendly and made terrible noises.

He saw some leaves on the ground. 'They can be my bed tonight,' he thought. 'Then I can decide what to do in the morning.' ⬛

❯

Toad jumps off the train it comes out the tunnel. H wants to run away from th people in the train behind. They want to take him bac to prison.

Think

Do you feel sorry for Toad? Why/ Why not?

[1] **tunnel** Look at the picture on page 47. The train is in a tunnel

Reading Comprehension

❶ Read the sentences and tick (✓) the ones you think are true.

☑ Toad didn't know where his friends were.

1 ☐ Toad's daughter came to visit him in prison.

2 ☐ Toad didn't eat any food.

3 ☐ Toad dressed in women's clothes.

4 ☐ At the station, Toad didn't have any money.

5 ☐ The train driver said that Toad could get on the train.

6 ☐ Toad jumped off the train at Toad Hall.

Reading

❷ Look at the picture on page 47 and answer the questions.

1 Is this an old or a new train?

2 How do you usually travel to school?

3 How do you usually travel when you go on holiday?

4 Are there many cars on the roads where you live?
Do you think this is good or bad? Why?

**21st
Century
Skills**

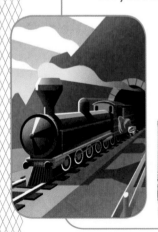

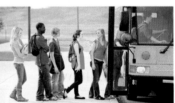

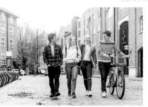

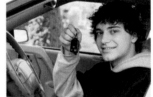

Reading and Writing MOVERS

3 **Look at the picture on page 47 again. Complete the sentences and answer the questions.**

The train is coming out of a ___tunnel___ .

1 What colour is the train? _____

2 Toad is wearing _____ .

3 How many wheels can you see? _____

4 What's Toad doing? _____

Writing

4 **Make some notes about Toad. What do you know about him now? Write four things.**

He lives in Toad Hall.

1 _____

2 _____

3 _____

4 _____

Before-reading Activities

Reading

5 **The next chapter is called, 'Here and There.'**
Why do you think it is called this? Read and see if you were right.

Listening

▶ 10 **6** **Listen to the first part of Chapter Five. Why is Rat unhappy?**

a ☐ Because Toad isn't there.

b ☐ Because he's bored.

c ☐ Because the birds are leaving.

Chapter 5

Here and There

▶10 Rat was unhappy, but he didn't know why. The summer was still[1] here. It was warm, and there was colour everywhere.

Then he looked at the birds, and he understood why he was unhappy.

It was time for the birds to leave and go somewhere else. ◼

▶11 'Do I want to be like them? Why do I feel unhappy? I have everything I need here,' he thought. But he could feel the sadness[2] in the air. He walked across the field and listened. He looked up to the sky. The sky was busy with birds flying here and there. Just[3] for a second, he wanted to be a bird.

Then he saw three birds on a tree, by the river.

'Hi, Rat!' they sang. 'Do you want to help us?'

'What are you doing?' asked Rat.

'We're leaving soon. We're making plans[4].'

'Why do you have to leave this lovely place?' asked Rat.

Rat is sad because summer is ending and for a moment he'd like to be like the birds who fly south, even if he loves where he lives.

Rat is talkin to the birds and he's sad because they're goin away.

---

[1] **still** until now
[2] **sadness** being sad
[3] **just** only
[4] **make plans** think about doing something

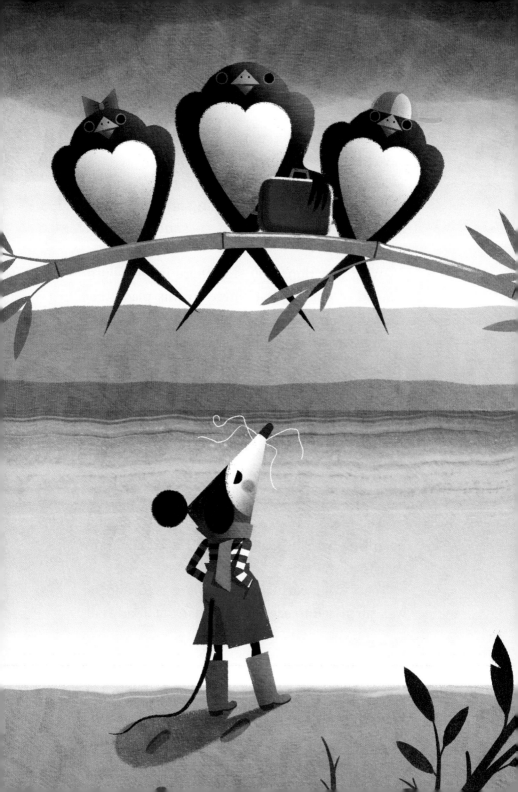

'You don't understand. We feel it inside. We have to go. We dream of it'.

'Can't you stay here? We're friends'.

'It's too cold, there's no sun and there aren't many insects[1]. We need to go south[2]! Oh, the south!'

'Well, why don't you stay there in the south, instead of coming back here to this place that you obviously[3] don't like very much at all?'

'Well, when we're in the south, this place begins to call us, too - the grass, the apple trees, the river and the insects. We miss[4] this place, too.'

Then the birds started talking amongst[5] themselves and forgot about Rat.

Rat walked on along the river: He looked towards[6] the south and had a strange feeling in his heart[7].

'The birds are going. Everything is changing, Toad isn't here' he thought. But Rat didn't know that Toad was very near.

Toad woke early. His feet were cold and he was surprised to see that he wasn't at Toad Hall,

---

[1] **insect**
[2] **south**
[3] **obviously** easy to understand
[4] **miss** when you think about a place you love and want to be there
[5] **amongst** in a group
[6] **towards** ➡
[7] **heart** ♥

in bed in his beautiful bedroom. He was cold. He was hungry. But he was free! Being free was like having fifty winter coats.

He brushed[1] his hair with his fingers[2], stood up, and then walked into the morning sun.

Toad got to the road, and started to look for somebody, anybody he could ask for directions[3]. He found a small river, and started to follow it.

Toad travelled for a long time, under the hot sun, when he saw a cart, and a man sitting there in front of a fire, making some food.

He looked at the man, and the man looked at him. But for a while[4] they didn't speak.

Then Toad said, 'Can you give me some of your food? I'm so hungry.'

'You can have some of my food,' said the man. 'But first you have to sing me a song. It gets lonely[5] out here on my own. And a song is just what I need.'

So Toad started to sing for his dinner. He sang a song about a brave and clever toad who had many friends. At first, Toad didn't want to sing, but when he started, he couldn't stop. He sang for

Toad is happy to be free but he's hungry snd wants to go home. He meets a man and asks him for some food. The man gives Toad something to eat after he sings for him.

---

[1] **brush** what you do to your hair with a hairbrush
[2] **finger** →
[3] **directions** the road to take
[4] **for a while** for some time
[5] **get lonely** how you feel when you have nobody to talk to

so long that after ten minutes the man said,

'Stop! That's enough.' He gave Toad some meat and potatoes.

When Toad was full[1] he said goodbye to the man, and he walked away happily, thinking about how clever he was. He started to sing another song. There was no one else[2] who could hear it, and again the song was about himself, and in the distance he saw something, something he knew well, something that excited him. He stopped singing, and then he heard a noise he loved.

Vroooooooommmmmmmmm!

'A car!' he said. 'I hope[3] I can get in.

Toad stood in the middle[4] of the road to stop the car and the car slowed down as it got near him. Toad's heart started to beat[5] fast. The excitement[6] was just too much.

'I love the car! I want it! I need it. No – Yes – No! Toad, be careful!' he said to himself.

And then Toad sat there in the road, crying.

The two people in the car got out, to look at this woman crying there in the middle of the road.

'The poor woman,' said one of the men.

Toad is still wearing women's clothes. He hears a car and he's excited. The men stop and put him in the car because they think Toad is an old woman crying because she's lost.

[1] **full** how you feel when you can't eat any more
[2] **no one else** no other people
[3] **hope** when you want something very much
[4] **middle** centre
[5] **beat** the noise your heart makes
[6] **excitement** when you feel happy because something is exciting

'She's probably[1] lost,' said the other man. 'Let's put her in our car, and take her where she wants to go.

Toad opened one eye. 'Thank you, kind gentlemen,' he said.

Then the men carried Toad into their car. He sat there in the back of the car, watching the road disappear in front of him.

'Can I sit in the front of the car?' said Toad.

'Of course,' said one of the men.

So Toad got into the front seat, and off they went again.

Toad was getting more and more excited.

'Please, Sir,' he said. 'Can I drive the car for a little while? It doesn't look difficult.'

The men laughed at what Toad said, 'Bravo, Madam! Why not? But drive carefully. Promise[2]?'

'I promise,' said Toad.

'Yes, I must be careful,' thought Toad. 'I just want to drive for a little while. Nice and slowly.'

At first Toad was careful. The car went slowly. But then he wanted to go faster, and faster and faster.

The gentlemen started to get worried. 'Be careful!' they both said.

[1] **probably** you say this when you think something but you don't know if you're right
[2] **to promise** to say that you are going to do something

Kenneth Grahame

Toad asks to drive the car and the men say yes. First, he drives slowly, then faster and faster. He crashes the car into the river. Then he runs away. He thinks he's so clever and starts to laugh but then he hears something...

Toad was angry at them for saying this, and he began to drive as fast as he could. 'I'm not an old woman,' he shouted. 'I'm Toad. Toad of Toad Hall. Sit still[1] and be quiet. You're about to learn what driving is. I'm Toad, the famous Toad.'

The men tried to stop Toad, but it was no use. The car went to the left, and then the right. And then ....

CRASH!!!

The car was no longer on the road. It was in the river and he was in the river, with the two gentlemen.

Toad got out of the water as quickly as he could, and ran and ran until he could run no more. When he began to feel better, he started to laugh.

'Oh, Toad! You're always the winner[2]! I got what I wanted again. I wanted to drive the car, and I did.'

Then he began to sing again.

'Oh, how clever I am! How clever, how clever, how very clev....'

But then he heard a noise in the distance. He turned to look and he saw... ◉

Think

Do you think Toad did the right thing?

[1] **sit still** don't move
[2] **winner** the best

Toad is driving too fast again!

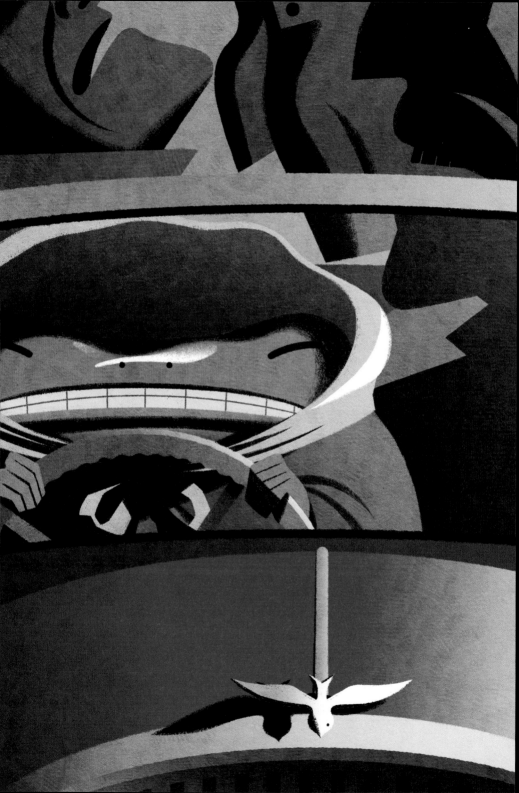

Reading and Writing

1 A **Read the sentences and decide who is speaking.**

> The man with a cart   The men in the car   Rat   Toad
> Rat   ~~The birds~~   Toad

We're leaving soon. We're making plans. _____The birds_____

1 Why do you have to go now? Can't you stay? _____

2 The birds are going. Everything is changing.
   Toad isn't here. _____

3 You can have some of my food, but first you have to sing
   me a song. _____

4 Can I sit in front of the car? _____

5 The poor woman, she's probably lost. _____

6 Oh, Toad! You're always the winner! _____

1 B **Read what Rat thinks about the birds and fill in the gaps.**

> ~~be~~ do feel need walked wanted was

Do I want to _____be_____ like them? Why (**1**) _____
I feel unhappy? I have everything I (**2**) _____ here,
he thought. But he could (**3**) _____ the sadness in the air,
and it (**4**) _____ difficult for him to be a normal and happy
Rat. He (**5**) _____ across the field and listened. He looked
up to the sky. The sky was busy with birds flying here and there.
Just for a second, he (**6**) _____ to be a bird.

Writing

21st
Century
Skills

2 **Rat says 'goodbye' to his friends, the birds.
They're leaving for another place. Where would you like
to go in the winter? Write a sentence.**

I would like to go to _____ because

_____ .

Reading and Writing MOVERS

3 **Choose the correct word for each sentence.**

Toad was surprised to see that he wasn't ___*at*___ Toad Hall.

~~at~~	to	on

1 He wanted to be _____ his bedroom.

to	in	at

2 He brushed his hair _____ his fingers.

by	from	with

3 He walked to the road to look _____ somebody.

for	at	up

4 Toad saw a man _____ a cart.

at	from	with

5 The man gave Toad some _____ his food.

of	with	by

6 Toad drove the car _____ the left and the right.

in	to	at

Before-reading Activities

Speaking

4 **The next chapter is called, 'Friends.' Why do you think it is called this?**

Listening

▶ 12 **5** **At the end of Chapter 5 what did Toad see? Listen to the first part of Chapter 6 to see if you are right.**

a ☐ His friends

b ☐ A car

c ☐ A train

Chapter 6

Friends

Toad runs away from the police but he falls into the river. The water is carrying him fast down the river but he pulls himself up onto the bank. Then he sees an animal. Who do you think it is?

12 Toad saw a car. Inside the car there were two policemen. Toad started to run again. 'Oh how silly I am, how silly I am,' he thought as he ran. ◼

13 He looked back, and saw that the car was getting nearer. He did his best but his legs were short and he couldn't run very fast. They were getting nearer and nearer, when suddenly he fell, and found himself once again in water. But this time the water moved fast, and it carried him away.

He couldn't stop the water, and he moved with it. He was going faster and faster, until he saw a tree. He put out his hands and held on to it for a few minutes and then slowly, he pulled himself up and out of the river and onto the bank.

Toad looked around and saw a dark hole. There was an animal inside. As the animal got nearer and nearer he saw a face; a brown face, with small ears and thick hair.

It was Rat!

Rat pulled Toad into his house. Toad was dirty and smelly[1], but happy to see his old friend.

'Oh, Rat,' he said. 'What a terrible, terrible time! I was in prison, but then I got out. I'm a clever toad. What do you think I did? I can't wait to tell you.'

'Toad!' said Rat. 'Stop talking now. Go upstairs and change into normal clothes[2]. Clean yourself, and try to look like a gentleman again. Stop talking and go! We can speak later.'

At first Toad was angry at Rat's words. 'People keep telling me what to do,' he thought. But then he saw himself in the mirror, and stopped being angry.

He changed his clothes and looked at the mirror again. 'How handsome[3] I am,' he thought.

When he came down, lunch was on the table and Toad was very glad[4] to see it. He was very hungry again. While Toad ate he started again to tell Rat how clever he was. But Rat said nothing.

When Toad stopped speaking, Rat said:

[1] **smelly**
[2] **normal clothes** what Toad usually wears
[3] **handsome** good-looking
[4] **glad** happy

'You're a really bad, Toad. When you see a car you forget everything else. You forget your friends. You think it's exciting, but don't you realise[1]? Do you think I'm happy to have a friend in prison?'

'You're right. I have to forget cars. I can buy a boat, a really fast boat instead.' Then he saw Rat's face.

'Ok, Rat, don't get angry[2] with me. It was only an idea. Let's drink our coffee and then we can walk to Toad Hall. I want to be sensible[3] now, Rat, I really do.'

'You want to walk to Toad Hall!' said Rat. 'You have no idea! This means that you don't know.'

'Don't know what?' asked Toad. 'What is it?'

'There are ferrets[4] living in Toad Hall now. Ferrets from the Wild Wood!'

'No!!!!!' shouted Toad. 'How? Why? When?' And then Toad started to cry.

'Tell me everything, dear Rat.'

'Well, when you went to prison, you disappeared for a time. Everyone knew about it, even the animals in the Wild Wood. The ferrets said 'He's never coming back, never! We tried to stop

Rat helps his friend again, but he's angry with Toad for being silly. Toad tells his friend that he wants to be a good toad now. Then Rat tells him that ferrets are now living at Toad Hall and Toad starts to cry.

Here's one of the ferret that are now living at Toa Hall. They came here when Toad was in priso Toad is very sad. How ca he get his house back?

[1] **realise** understand
[2] **be angry** feel bad about what someone does
[3] **sensible** a sensible person doesn't do silly things
[4] **ferrets** see picture on page 63

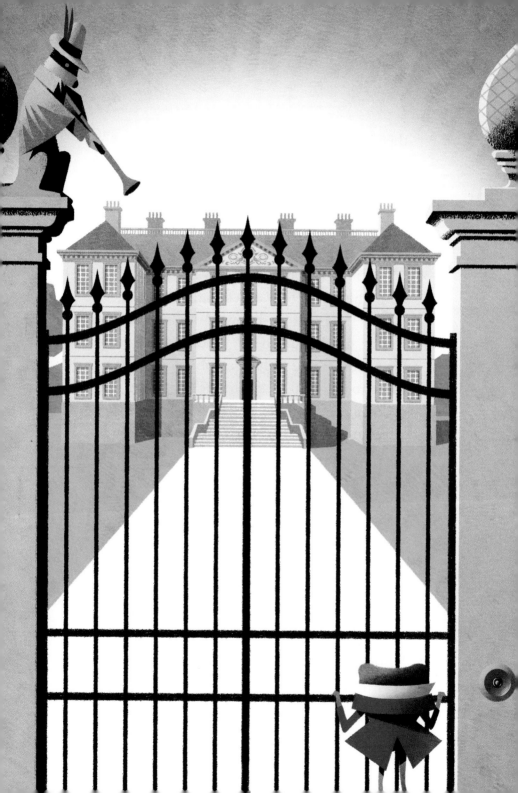

them, but they moved in[1] and made themselves very comfortable.'

'The ferrets lie[2] in bed all day, and eat all the time, and never clean the house. They sing rude[3] songs about you. They tell everybody that they want to stay there forever.'

'No, no, they can't stay in my house!' said Toad.

'It's no good, Toad,' called Rat. 'You can't get in.'

But Toad was on his way[4] to Toad Hall. He walked quickly down the road, with a stick[5] in his hand, talking to himself about what he was going to do, until he got to the front gate, when suddenly he saw a big ferret with a gun[6].

'Who is it?' said the Ferret.

'What do you mean by talking to me like that,' said Toad angrily.

Then he heard a noise

BANG.

Toad ran back down the road. He could hear the ferret laughing.

When Toad got back to Rat's house, Mole and Badger were there too.

Toad is angry and wants to tell the ferrets to go away from his home. But when he gets to Toad Hall, one of the ferrets has a gun. Toad is afraid and runs back to Rat's house.

[1] **move in** go and live in a house
[2] **lie** stay
[3] **rude** not nice
[4] **was on his way** was going
[5] **stick** ⌐_____
[6] **gun** what the ferret is holding in picture 63

'Welcome home, Toad,' said Badger.

'Hooray! Here's Toad,' said Mole. 'You're a clever animal. You got out of prison.'

Toad started to feel happy and clever again. But then he remembered his poor friends. They were really worried about him.

After dinner, Rat, Mole and Badger told Toad about Toad Hall.

'It seems impossible to get in. There are so many ferrets,' said Rat. 'But, we have an idea.'

'Now for the first time in your life you must listen to your friends,' said Badger. 'Toad, you don't know this, your father never told you. There's a tunnel. It starts near the river and goes right into the middle of Toad Hall. There's a big party tomorrow night for all the ferrets.'

'While they're having their party, we can go through the tunnel that takes us to the kitchen,' said Mole.

'Let's rest,' said Rat. 'We have to be strong tomorrow, to get Toad's house back.'

The next day, when it was dark, the animals got

Rat, Mole and Badger want to help their friend Toad to get his house back from the ferrets. They can get into the house through a tunnel that goes from the river to the kitchen in Toad Hall.

ready for the adventure. Badger took a lamp and said, "follow me". They walked silently towards the river. Soon they were at the beginning of the tunnel. It was cold and dark, and Toad was getting really frightened.

'Help me!' said Toad.

'Be quiet, Toad, or we must leave you behind,' said Badger.

The four friends moved through the tunnel slowly until at last Badger said, 'We're nearly under Toad's house now.' They could hear ferrets above their heads - ferrets having a party.

They started to walk,

Up!

Up!

Up!

and soon they arrived at[1] a door – the door that took them into the kitchen.

They opened the door and went up into the kitchen, and then they listened to the ferrets.

The ferrets were dancing to music, and

---

[1] **arrive at** come to

laughing. It was too much for Toad. He rushed[1] into the room with his friends.

The ferrets knew how to have a party, but they weren't very brave. They ran away as soon as they saw Rat, Mole, Badger and Toad. They jumped out of the window, up the chimney[2], anywhere to get away from an angry Toad.

After five minutes there were no more ferrets. They all ran towards the river, and Toad Hall was once again Toad's house.

The next morning, Toad came down late for breakfast as usual. Mole and Rat were sitting out in the garden. Badger was in an armchair reading the newspaper.

Badger looked up, 'We have a lot of work to do this morning. We want to have a big party to celebrate our victory[3].'

'Oh, all right,' said Toad. 'Anything you want. But can I sing just one song at the party?'

'No,' said Badger. 'No more songs and silly games. You have to change now.'

The four friends get into Toad Hall through the tunnel. The ferrets aren't brave and they run away when they see how angry Toad is.

---

[1] **rush** go quickly
[2] **chimney** 🏭
[3] **celebrate our victory** have a party because they're happy that they sent the ferrets away

'Very well. I promise to be a very different Toad from now on.'

It was a very good party. So many animals came to welcome Toad back. But when they asked him for a song, or a story about himself, he said.

'No, this is not the time for songs. This is the time to say how lucky I am to have such good friends.'

Rat, Mole, Badger and Toad sat around the table, and looked at each other and smiled.

Friends forever!

Toad promises to be good and he's very happy to have such good friends.

Toad and all his friends have a party. They're happy that Toad is back in his house again.

Think

How important is to have good friends?

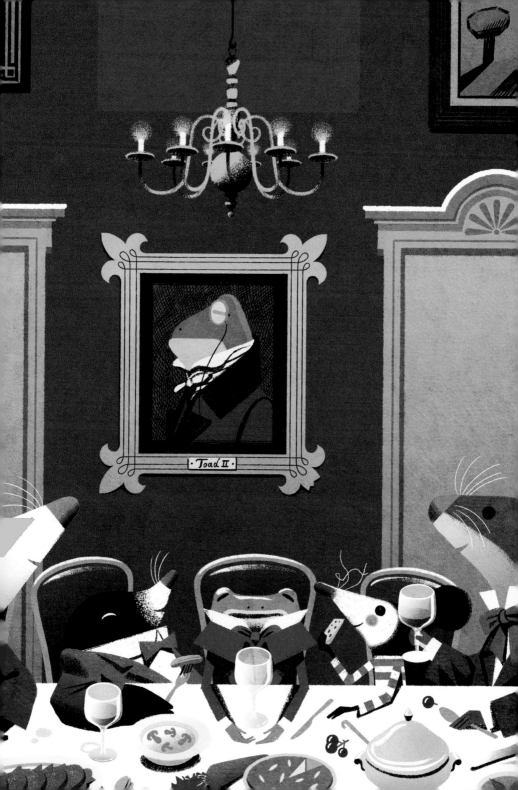

Reading Comprehension

1 **Number these sentences in the order that they happen in Chapter 6.**

a ☐ Rat, Mole, Badger and Toad get into Toad Hall.
b ☐ Toad goes to Toad Hall alone.
c ☐ Toad sees Mole and Badger again.
d ☐1 Toad is in the water.
e ☐ Toad and his friends have a party.
f ☐ Toad sees Rat.

Speaking and Writing

2 **In the story, Rat, Badger and Mole help Toad many times. They're good friends. Discuss these questions with a partner, then write your answers.**

21st Century Skills

1 How do you help your friends?
_____

2 What do you look for in a friend?
_____

3 What do you like doing with your friends?
_____

4 Why is it important to have friends?
_____

5 Do you prefer a big group of friends or just one best friend? Why?
_____

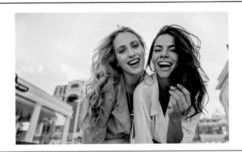

Speaking

3 **Which chapter of the story did you like the most? Why?**

☐ Chapter 1 *My World*
☐ Chapter 2 *The Wild Wood*
☐ Chapter 3 *Home*
☐ Chapter 4 *Run Toad Run!*
☐ Chapter 5 *Here and There*
☐ Chapter 6 *Friends*

Vocabulary

4 **Put the words in the box into the correct category.**
Use the table below. Then write any other words you know.

bird boat biscuits cart horse jam mole
orange juice train snow sun wind

1 Animals	
2 Food	
3 Transport	
4 Weather	

Reading and Writing   **MOVERS**

5 **Look at the picture on page 69. Complete the sentences**
and answer the questions.

There is a picture of Toad on the _____*wall.*_____ .
1 What colour is Mole's jacket? _____
2 Toad is wearing a white _____ .
3 How many carrots can you see? _____
4 What's Rat doing? _____

Kenneth Grahame

Kenneth Grahame
Born on 8 March 1859 in Edinburgh, Scotland.

1858

Family
His mother died when Grahame was only five years old. Grahame, his two brothers and his sister went to live with their grandmother in the countryside of Berkshire. This place gave him ideas for his famous book *The Wind in the Willows*.

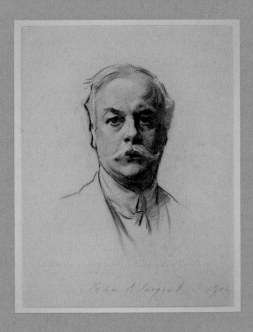

Early life
He started school at the age of nine and was a good student. He didn't go to university because his family didn't have enough money. Instead, he started to work in a bank in London.

Early works
He started to write when he moved to London, first, for magazines, then, a collection of short stories called *The Golden Age*. In 1898, he wrote another collection of stories called Dream Days.

1898

1909

1929

The Wind in the Willows

His book was so popular that Grahame could stop working in the bank and he went back to the countryside. In 1929, the writer A. A. Milne wrote a play for the theatre called *Toad of Toad Hall*. Later, Disney made a film of Grahame's book.

The book is still popular with children today.

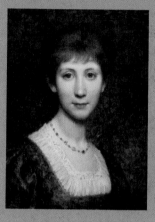

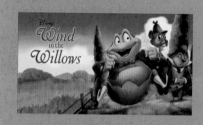

Personal life

He married Elspeth Thomson in 1899. They had one child, a boy called Alastair, who was often very ill. Grahame told his son stories at bedtime about a Toad and Alastair loved them. These same stories later became the book *The Wind in the Willows* in October 1908. Alastair died when he was only twenty, and after losing his son, Grahame didn't write very much.

1899

1932

Last years

After his son died, Grahame lived in Oxford with his wife until he died on 6 July 1932.

Rat, Mole, Badger and Toad

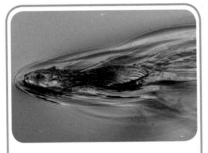

Rat

Rat is actually a water rat. He's different from normal rats because he knows how to swim. In fact, he's very good at swimming. He doesn't usually like large groups and prefers to live alone. He's a dark brown colour, and he has small ears and a round face. He's quite big and can grow up to 22 centimetres long. He likes eating plants and fruit and doesn't eat meat. He eats a lot. In the winter he lives in a hole, but he always has to be close to the water. Sadly, he doesn't live for a very long time - normally only two years. Many other animals, like birds, think that the water rat is very good to eat. Life isn't easy for our friend, Rat.

Mole

Mole is a very shy animal. He's very small, and lives in a tunnel. He likes to eat insects, and is very good at finding places to keep food when he's hungry. A mole can smell things from very far away. In the story, Mole smells his home.

Like the water rat, the mole doesn't live very long. He usually lives for four years. Many other animals want to eat moles. That's why they stay inside their tunnel most of the time.

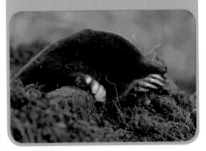

Now you know the characters in the story, what do you know about these animals? They're very interesting creatures. Here are some interesting facts about them.

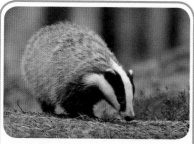

Badger

The badger has a short body and short legs which he uses to find food and make tunnels. His colours are black, brown, gold and white. He can grow up to 51 to 86 centimetres long from head to tail, and his tail can be 10 to 15 cm long. He usually sleeps during the day, and is awake at night.

He's a very clean animal and likes to live with other badgers. He eats both plants and insects. Sometimes he gets very sleepy and can sleep for days or weeks in his home. He lives a little bit longer than the water rat and the mole - for about 10 years.

Toad

The toad is a type of frog. He has very short legs and hard skin. He's different from frogs because he doesn't jump as much. He prefers to walk. A toad's skin doesn't taste very nice. For this reason, not many animals want to eat him. In fact, if you touch a toad, wash your hands afterwards.

A toad can grow up to 18 centimetres long. He likes wet places but doesn't have to be near a river. He likes to eat insects, spiders and worms, and he usually eats at night.

A toad prefers to live on his own. He lives much longer than the water rat, the mole and the badger - sometimes for twenty to forty years.

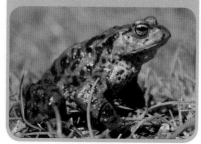

Getting Around

Toad really enjoys driving his car.
A car was a really special thing 100 years ago.
Today we see cars all the time, but when
Kenneth Grahame wrote,
'The Wind in the Willows',
it was quite rare to see
a car on the road.
How did most
people get around
in the early 1900s?
Read and see.

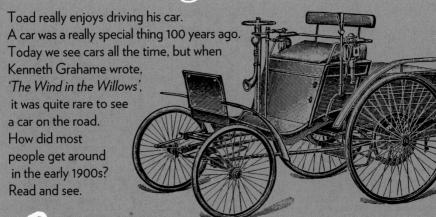

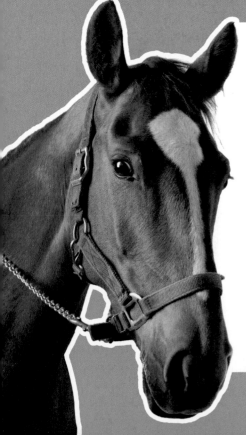

The Horse

In 1900, most people used horses to
move from one place to another. The
streets were not full of cars, but full of
horses. In the story we can see that a
horse pulled Toad's cart. Travelling
by horse was much more difficult than
travelling by train or car. A horse can
travel about 40 miles in a day, if the road
is good. But often the roads weren't good
and so the distance was much shorter.

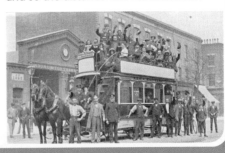

The Car

There were very few cars at this time, and they were only for very rich people (or rich Toads!). In 1895, there were only 14 or 15 cars in the whole of Britain. Seeing a motor car on the road was very strange and very exciting. The cars were beautifully made and looked very nice. Many people who had cars didn't know how to drive. They had a driver who took them around. When 'The Wind in the Willows' became popular, the Ford Model T was invented. They were the first cars that were cheap enough for people to buy. This type of car arrived in Britain in 1911. After this, there were a lot more cars on the roads.

The Train

For longer distances, people used trains. A train could take people from one part of the country to another. Trains in those times were very noisy, and people could hear them when they were near. That's why Toad knew there was a train coming when he got out of prison. Trains carried people and sometimes things to be sold. Early trains were much slower than modern trains.

In Britain, where the story takes place, the railway system was very important, and you could even go from one small village to another by train.

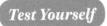

Answer the questions with the names of the characters in the box.

Badger   Mole   Rat   Toad

Who:

	has no money to buy a train ticket?	_Toad_
1	has a boat?	_____
2	dresses in an old woman's clothes?	_____
3	lives in the Wild Wood?	_____
4	can't swim?	_____
5	sings songs?	_____
6	says goodbye to the birds?	_____
7	does Badger get angry with?	_____
8	tells Toad about the tunnel?	_____
9	leaves his house when it's dirty?	_____
10	goes to prison?	_____
11	smells his home?	_____
12	has a big house?	_____
13	loves the river?	_____
14	has a green door?	_____
15	wants to go nowhere with Rat?	_____
16	sleeps a lot?	_____
17	goes out alone in the Wild Wood?	_____
18	buys a car?	_____
19	tells Toad about the Ferrets?	_____
20	knows everything about the Wild Wood?	_____

Vocabulary Areas
Animals
Food
Transport
Weather
Nature

Tags
Animals
Friendship
Adventure
Nature

Grammar and Structures
Present simple: states and habits
Present continuous: actions in progress
Past simple: past actions in a finished time
Can: ability, request
Could: past form of *can; must* - obligation; *have to* - necessity
Adverbs; comparative and superlative adjectives; prepositions
(place, time); question words
Relative clauses
There is/There are
Pronouns
verbs + infinitive/*-ing*

Teen **ELi** Readers

Stage 1
Maureen Simpson, *In Search of a Missing Friend*
Charles Dickens, *Oliver Twist*
Geoffrey Chaucer, *The Canterbury Tales*
Janet Borsbey & Ruth Swan, *The Boat Race Mystery*
Lucy Maud Montgomery, *Anne of Green Gables*
Mark Twain, *A Connecticut Yankee in King Arthur's Court*
Mark Twain, *The Adventures of Huckleberry Finn*
Angela Tomkinson, *Great Friends!*
Edith Nesbit, *The Railway Children*
Eleanor H. Porter, *Pollyanna*
Anna Sewell, *Black Beauty*
Kenneth Grahame, *The Wind in the Willows*

Stage 2
Elizabeth Ferretti, *Dear Diary...*
Angela Tomkinson, *Loving London*
Mark Twain, *The Adventures of Tom Sawyer*
Mary Flagan, *The Egyptian Souvenir*
Maria Luisa Banfi, *A Faraway World*
Frances Hodgson Burnett, *The Secret Garden*
Robert Louis Stevenson, *Treasure Island*
Elizabeth Ferretti, *Adventure at Haydon Point*
William Shakespeare, *The Tempest*
Angela Tomkinson, *Enjoy New York*
Frances Hodgson Burnett, *Little Lord Fauntleroy*
Michael Lacey Freeman, *Egghead*
Michael Lacey Freeman, *Dot to Dot*
Silvana Sardi, *The Boy with the Red Balloon*
Silvana Sardi, *Scotland is Magic!*
Silvana Sardi, *Garpur: My Iceland*
Silvana Sardi, *Follow your Dreams*
Gabriele Rebagliati, *Naoko: My Japan*

Stage 3
Anna Claudia Ramos, *Expedition Brazil*
Charles Dickens, *David Copperfield*
Mary Flagan, *Val's Diary*
Maureen Simpson, *Destination Karminia*
Anonymous, *Robin Hood*
Jack London, *The Call of the Wild*
Louisa May Alcott, *Little Women*
Gordon Gamlin, *Allan: My Vancouver*

Kenneth Grahame
The Wind in the Willows

Toad is never happy to sit at home and do nothing. He likes adventure and fun. Sometimes things go wrong, but he is a lucky Toad. He has the most important thing that anyone can have.

He has friends. He has Rat, and Mole, and Badger. Follow these four friends around the English countryside. Visit them inside their houses, and travel with them in a car, or on a boat on the river. Listen to the Wind in the Willows.

In this reader you will find:
- Information about Kenneth Grahame
- A section focusing on background and context
- A glossary of difficult words
- Comprehension and grammar activities including
  A1 Movers style exercises and 21st century skills activities
- Final test

Tags
Adventure | Nature | Friendship

 Look at the inside front cover flap to find out how to download your free Audio files.

● **STAGE 1**	**600 headwords**	**Elementary**	**A1**	**Movers**
STAGE 2	800 headwords	Pre-intermediate	A2	Flyers/Key
STAGE 3	1000 headwords	Intermediate	B1	Preliminary

Classic

www.eligradedreaders.com

Eli Readers is a beautifully illustrated series of timeless classic and original stories for learners of English.

ELI *The pleasure of Reading*

ISBN 978-88-536-3191-6